A WORKING FAITH

A WORKING FAITH

*Essays and Addresses on
Science, Medicine and Ethics*

by

JOHN HABGOOD
Bishop of Durham

Darton, Longman & Todd
London

First published in Great Britain in 1980 by
Darton, Longman & Todd Ltd
89 Lillie Road, London SW6 1UD

© 1980 John Habgood

ISBN 0 232 51454 2

Printed in Great Britain by The Anchor Press Ltd
and bound by Wm Brendan & Son Ltd
both of Tiptree, Essex

CONTENTS

Introduction

Part One: Science and Faith

Part Two: The Ethical Dimension in Science and Technology

Part Three: Medical Ethics

To ROSALIE

INTRODUCTION

The strength of the Christian movement depends upon its capacity to generate a vocabulary of symbols which could be co-ordinated to cover all the contingencies of human existence. Its power would be demonstrated if there was no deep concern of the human psyche which could not respond to the Gospel, and no lofty aspiration of the Spirit which it could not irradiate. . . .[1]

In this rather alarming quotation Bruce Reed sets a standard for Christian faith, which anyone seriously committed to it dare not refuse. To make claims about God is potentially to say something about everything. If this were not so, then the God Christians talk about would not be the Lord of all life, and the source and ground of all existence.

I emphasize the word 'potentially', because in practice most of human life has to be lived without conscious reference to God and, even in the most religious people, with only a general background awareness of his presence. Nevertheless the potentiality is there. Events, objects, insights, choices, can be illuminated by faith; and the test of a faith that works is that it should constantly be capable of providing this kind of illumination.

At first sight there is an absurd contrast between Christian claims to universality and the narrow base on which Christianity actually rests. The National Library of Congress receives nine thousand new books every day; the New Testament contains about three hundred pages. When all the

1. *The Dynamics of Religion* (D.L.T. 1978), p. 220.

usual things have been said about quantity and quality, the
assertion that this little book somehow contains the decisive
clues to the significance of human life, seems either stagger-
ingly impudent or deplorably short-sighted. The sum of
human knowledge and experience covers such a vast range
that it is hardly surprising when the word 'God', understood
in its universal implications, dies on many people's lips.

In calling this book *A Working Faith*, I have this contrast in
mind. I have not attempted to write systematically about
theology, nor to set out my personal faith in anything but the
most oblique and incoherent fashion. My aim has been to try
to demonstrate what happens when a fairly conventional
Christian believer tries to *work with* faith in facing the
demands, conflicts, and questions which arise in particular,
fairly circumscribed, areas of human experience. Universal
claims for the Christian faith have to be defended on the basis
of broad generalizations about the nature of God and the
mode of his self-revelation. But the defence can only begin to
be plausible if here and there it can be shown in some detail
that belief in the Christian revelation actually makes a difference. To use the current jargon, large theological statements
have to be cashed at every available local check-out point.

By 'a working faith', then, I mean a faith which is put to
work in tackling many different issues, which may by themselves seem marginal to the central Christian beliefs, but
which together represent something of the complexity, inter-
connectedness, and recalcitrance of the world in which faith
has to be exercised. In other words, we can only test whether
the Christian 'vocabulary of symbols' covers 'all the contingencies of human existence' by actually trying it out in the
contingencies which face us. Local successes do not prove the
larger claim. But they can make it seem less arrogant.

An analogy may help. In all the millions of books in the
National Library of Congress, how many basic themes are
there? Scientific knowledge, despite the huge complexity of its
detail, depends in the last resort on a comparatively small
number of key concepts. The same is true of the world of

nature. Seemingly endless variety has arisen through ringing the changes on a simple genetic code. To say this is not to deny the complexity; it is merely to point out that it can co-exist with simplicity. There may in fact be nodal points in human experience, centrally important ideas and insights, of which it is not absurd to claim that they have a universal significance. The claim can only be supported, however, as again and again such nodal points prove their importance in the actual business of coping with detail.

All this may seem a somewhat portentous way of introducing a book of occasional essays and addresses. Bishops are always talking on this or that, and nobody except God checks up on whether they are being consistent. But if, at the heart of all this activity, there is a faith which is actually doing some useful work, then it seems to me that a case study of the way in which one Christian has tried to tackle a variety of concrete problems may be of some interest. My hope is that the problems are of interest in themselves. However, in this introduction I am more concerned to draw attention to the general approach which underlies them.

Cross-fertilization is not a bad name for it. I have been lucky enough to work in three very different kinds of professional environment. As a young research student in the Cambridge Physiological Laboratory during one of its great periods I gained, and I hope have never lost, a strong awareness of the assumptions, attitudes, and feelings which underlie scientific work, and which are almost impossible to convey in a formal description of scientific method. As a teacher of theology, often having to deal with students who had taken a first degree in science, I was constantly reminded of the very different world which a theologian can seem to inhabit. As a member of a family in which medicine extends over five generations, and as a teacher of medical students myself, I have been immersed in the concerns and atmosphere of the medical profession for most of my life.

My aim has been to keep these different worlds together. This is more than an exercise in defining boundaries. The frontiers between different disciplines are usually the places of greatest interest, and also the greatest danger. Multi-disciplinary studies can be marvellously fertile or notoriously sloppy. I do not pretend to have escaped the dangers. But I believe I have witnessed enough genuine cross-fertilization to be able to say that in the little bit of the world I inhabit, the universal claims of the Christian faith ring true.

Cross-fertilization works both ways. The extent to which scientific understanding has brought new insights into, and in some respects changed the character of, theology is part of the intellectual history of the last three hundred years. My essay on Darwin is an attempt to map one small section of that history. The one on *Computerized Values* looks at the way in which the behavioural sciences are beginning to have an impact on ethics. Other essays pre-suppose that theology and ethics must take scientific knowledge into account.

The reverse process is harder to identify. Scientists are on the whole deeply jealous of the autonomy of their subject, and some are suspicious of any suggestion that it might have frontiers at all, let alone ones across which useful contributions might flow. Yet increasingly in recent years this isolationism has been broken down. Scientists have to live in the real world in which complex issues of social and personal behaviour cannot be avoided. They are asked to advise on numerous practical issues which are not amenable to the rigorous kind of scientific analysis which has won such successes in the fields of physics, chemistry, and biology. They have had to face questions about the values which sustain science, and the responsibility of scientists for the uses to which their work is put. And sometimes the very heartlands of scientific theory have been invaded by those who point to hidden assumptions about meaning and the nature of scientific understanding.

W. H. Pannenberg's major work *Theology and the Philosophy of Science*.[2] is a notable modern example of this latter, rather

2. D.L.T. 1976.

rarified, approach. I tried to spell out some of its implications in my radio talk *Truth and Dr Steiner*, in response to a very curious broadcast by Dr Steiner, which seemed to me to represent scientific isolationism at its worst.

The main area of cross-fertilization in this direction, however, is in the field of ethics and social responsibility, and Christians still have a gigantic task to do in shaping a theology which can give some real insights into what on earth we ought to be doing with all our scientific and technological expertise. The World Council of Churches has given a good lead through its studies on Church and Society. Its 1979 Conference on *Science, Faith and the Future* brought together scientists and theologians from all over the world to explore these themes, and my sermon to it, 'Be like God', was an attempt to provide a simple theological focus for the multitude of conflicting topics which the Conference tried to cover.

Medical ethics has progressed much further than ethical thinking in other branches of science. It is not at all uncommon to find articles on particular ethical issues rubbing shoulders with straightforward research papers in medical literature, in a way which would still seem very surprising in a more strictly scientific journal. No doubt this is partly because medicine is only scientific in some of its aspects. Those whose science is so immediately and intimately related to the well-being of individuals cannot afford to neglect the ethical dimension in their work. It is interesting, however, that the more scientific medicine becomes, the sharper the ethical dilemmas it provokes. There could well be a parallel between this and the growing concern about social responsibility in science, now that the power of scientific advances to change the whole fabric of human life has been so alarmingly demonstrated.

Be that as it may, medicine has accumulated an impressive ethical tradition, so much so that it is possible for those who write about particular problems to be reasonably confident that their contribution is welcomed and their assumptions broadly accepted. Many of the essays in this book fall into this category and since, on the whole, they were prepared for medical, rather than specifically Christian, consumption, the religious basis on which they rest is not made explicit. Clergy have an advantage in that their Christian assumptions are, whether justifiably or not, usually taken for granted by their audiences.

The two articles on Spina Bifida are examples of the kind of papers produced by a small medical group in Newcastle, of which I am the Chairman and chief draftsman. They have been shortened by the removal of some of the more technical material, and have been included because the experience of preparing them in a multi-disciplinary group has for me provided a vivid illustration of cross-fertilization at work. Teasing one's way through severely practical problems, about which life and death decisions have to be made, is a good reminder that finding a faith to live by is not merely an academic exercise.

I am grateful, therefore, to those who have prodded me by their invitations to write the various pieces which make up this book. I am conscious that it comes nowhere near answering the challenge of my opening quotation. But I hope it may encourage others to go on trying.

PART ONE
SCIENCE AND FAITH

1
AFTER DARWIN

There is a stage in the development of some major scientific theories when they cease to be regarded as theories and become unquestioned assumptions underlying a whole branch of science. This is now the status of the theory of evolution. Without it modern biology would be a shambles. In fact it is no exaggeration to say that it was Darwin who transformed the study of natural history into the science of biology by providing it with its key explanatory concept. The most striking characteristic of living organisms is that they appear to adapt themselves purposefully to their environment. Darwin explained this power of adaptation by the simple insight that only those organisms best adapted to live in their environment do in fact survive. In every example of biological adaptation the fruitful question to ask was no longer 'What purpose does this fulfil?' but 'What advantage does it give its possessor in the struggle for existence?' The difference may seem small, but it marks the transition from an early phase of science, which is mainly descriptive, to the phase of main scientific advance, which is explanatory and experimental; from a partly subjective phase, to a wholly objective one. Once this phase in a science has been reached, and has proved its fruitfulness, it becomes unthinkable ever to go back to the earlier one. There may be subsequent modifications in the key concepts; there may even be scientific revolutions; but the key concepts cannot be denied without destroying the science itself.

This chapter was originally published in *The Expository Times* in Jan. 1973 as 'They changed our thinking: Pt. 1, Darwin and After'.

I make this point briefly and dogmatically because there are still some Christians who try to protect themselves against what they regard as scientific threats to their faith by reiterating that evolution is 'only a theory'. Any Christian who has the temerity to bradcast on the subject of evolution usually finds himself bombarded afterwards with anti-evolutionist literature. But beyond the lunatic fringe, there seem to be countless believers who have not yet fully and gladly accepted what biology has to tell us about ourselves, and who perhaps vaguely hope that somehow the scientists have got it all wrong. This is a delusion. Though scientists are certainly not infallible, and though sciences change and develop, it cannot be stated too clearly that evolution is not a theory which might be upset by contrary evidence tomorrow or the day after; it is the only conceivable basis for modern biology. In fact, the general idea of evolution is more than this. To see the universe, not as a collection of static fragments, but as a developing and explicable whole, has involved a revolution in human consciousness within the last hundred years, a revolution in which Darwin played a central role; and this, too, would be in jeopardy if evolution were 'only a theory'. As Teilhard de Chardin put it, 'What makes and classifies a "modern" man (and a whole host of our contemporaries is not yet "modern" in this sense) is having become capable of seeing in terms not of space and time alone, but also of duration, or – and it comes to the same thing – of biological space-time; and above all having become incapable of seeing anything otherwise – anything – *not even himself.*'[1]

Of course, it was not always so. In the beginning Darwin's theory had to fight for its life, and we must not be too hard on our Christian forefathers in their opposition to it. There were then good scientific reasons for doubting its adequacy, and it was not until the rediscovery of Mendel's work on genetics in 1900 that the most serious difficulty was overcome. There have been many changes of emphasis since Darwin's

1. Teilhard de Chardin, *The Phenomenon of Man* (1959), p. 219.

day, and modern evolutionary theory is very different from
and far more sophisticated than early Darwinism. But what
kept it alive during the lean years was the recognition that,
inadequacies or no, this was the right kind of explanation to
look for if biology was ever to be rescued from its former
dependence on theology, and that there was in fact no
alternative.

Darwin's work had not been done in a vacuum. Evolutionary ideas had been current long before his day. The concept
of natural selection had been arrived at independently by
Wallace at about the same time, a fact which eventually
forced the reluctant Darwin to publish. It is not belittling his
genius to say that if he had not written *The Origin of Species*
somebody else would have done so. There seems, in short, to
be a momentum in scientific advance which, while not dispensing with the crucially important work of individuals,
makes particular periods ripe for particular kinds of discovery.
It is thus possible for scientists to feel in their bones that
something must be right, even if the evidence for it is not
watertight. With theologians, on the other hand, feeling in
their bones that evolutionary theory struck at the root of their
doctrine of man, the stage was set for a conflict which was
not, repeat not, a mere instance of ecclesiastical dogmatism
versus scientific enlightenment, but in which respectable
scientific arguments could be mustered on both sides. A lot
of the controversy was, of course, disreputable and ridiculous.
But that there was a solid core of doubt is attested by the fact
that even in our own day there are leading theologians who
try to blur the edges of evolutionary theory and escape its full
implications. I remember hearing Charles Raven, than whom
no one was more scathing in his denunciation of scientific
unenlightenment, draw the line at the evolution of the cuckoo
and claim that here, at any rate, in its complex life style
something more than natural selection was required. And
which of us does not add all sorts of mental reservations when
we think about the evolution of man?

But the fact is that during the last hundred years, Darwin's basic ideas have been vindicated again and again. In the last twenty, the molecular basis of evolutionary change has begun to be revealed, and there are now no adequate scientific grounds for opposition. This is something which, I believe, theologians ought gladly and gratefully to accept, as marking the end of a rather miserable chapter in their relationships with science. I shall try to justify this opinion later. Meanwhile, it is important to notice the differences between present-day evolutionary theory and early Darwinism. While not affecting the fundamental issues, some of these have changed the feel of the theory so that it seems less sharply antagonistic to belief in a loving Providence.

First, and most important, has been the development of genetics already mentioned, and in particular the discovery of mutations. It is now possible to give a precise meaning to the notion of individual variation within species, which Darwin recognized as the material upon which natural selection works. We now know in considerable biochemical detail how the shuffling of the genes takes place, how sexual reproduction can be a source of almost infinite variety, what is the physical basis of individual identity, and why it is possible to predict that every now and then there should be sudden evolutionary leaps. All this has immensely strengthened the original theory, and has enabled the kind of mathematical predictions to be made which demonstrate that what biologists claim must have happened is statistically possible.

Secondly, the emphasis in the theory has shifted away from the notion of the isolated individual locked in a life and death struggle against all other organisms, towards that of the population, or 'gene pool', as the evolving entity. Species, in other words, evolve as wholes. And more than that, they evolve in relation to other species so that what is eventually attained is a balance, a mutuality, often a high degree of co-operation and interdependence. Our present concern with ecology should have brought home to us that the so-called law of the jungle is actually a very complex, delicately adjusted law, of which 'nature red in tooth and claw' is a travesty. This is not to deny that creatures kill each other. Death is a necessary consequence of reproduction. But the only creature which wantonly kills its own kind appears to be man.

Thirdly, one of the most powerful creative factors in evolution is seen to be environmental change. In a stable environment the 'struggle for existence' leads to the kind of balance just described. Only under conditions of stress do small physical improvements or behavioural changes become important. The primitive fishes which left the lakes and experimented with life on land started a new evolutionary era as the lakes dried up. Their response to stress gave them a decisive advantage. If the lakes had remained as they were, the land could well have remained uncolonized.

What this implies in general is that the evolutionary process favours adaptability. In a world where disasters can happen there is a built-in advantage for those creatures which are either so simple as to be relatively impervious to change, or so complex as to be able to respond to new circumstances in new ways. Which, to cut a very long story short, is probably why the most successful species on earth are bacteria and men.

Fourthly, since Darwin's day it has become evident that behavioural change may be as important as structural change in ensuring the success of a species. For example, a bird gains no advantage by having a longer beak than others unless it searches for food in places which are inaccessible to its short-beaked brothers. Structure and function are inter-connected. An understanding of evolution, therefore, which concentrates solely on physical, and in particular genetic, change, and makes no allowance for the way animals actually behave, is grossly one-sided. Not all biologists are equally convinced about the importance of this factor, but if accepted it points to the same general conclusions as in the previous example. In an evolutionary process where behaviour counts, there is a tendency to favour inquiring, exploratory, and ultimately intelligent organisms. This may be the truth behind Teilhard de Chardin's claim that evolution has a direction, a favoured axis, coinciding with the development of man. The form in which he often presented this thesis was unconvincing and has won little support among scientists. But at least it can be plausibly argued that the advent of intelligence on earth was not a mere accident, however much accident may have entered into the process whereby it came to be.

A fifth development worth mentioning concerns the degree to which evolutionary concepts have been extended outside the realm of biological evolution. This is a complex story about which there are wide differences of opinion. It is possible, I believe, to distinguish very roughly between an earlier illegitimate phase in which it was assumed that the mechanism of evolution was in some sense universally operative, and a later much more acceptable phase in which the idea of evolution has been immensely fruitful, but the various means whereby it happens have been regarded as distinct. Social Darwinism, for instance, assumed that the forces of natural selection ought to be allowed to operate unimpeded within society, and thus formed a powerful ally for *laissez-faire* economics; it has rightly been discredited. Nevertheless it is perfectly proper to study the evolution of society, and even to talk about the natural selection of those institutions and customs fitted to survive, provided it is recognized that the explanation of social development is not and cannot be the same as the explanation of biological development, because the methods of transmission of the social and biological inheritances from one generation to another are totally and fundamentally different. This reminder is needed as a warning both to those who talk too easily about the evolution of this, that or the other, and to those who unreasonably resist language about, say, the evolution of the soul, or the evolution of ideas, or the evolution of ethics through fear that the word somehow explains them away. Evolution, as I have said earlier, is an all-embracing concept which is here to stay. But it does not follow from this that the natural selection of inherited variables is an all-embracing explanation.

These five developments in evolutionary theory could well

be superseded by others of even greater significance for theology, since no theory is ever fixed or final despite the apparent unshakability of its central concepts. But in themselves they add up to a considerable shift of emphasis. Nor has theology stood still in the interim. In some respects, therefore, the modern theologian in coming to terms with Darwinism has a different task from that of his predecessors. Genesis is no longer an issue. With Adam occupying his proper mythological status there seems no good reason to insist that humanity must have begun with a single pair, or even at a definite time. Nor need the doctrine of the Fall have an historical basis, except in the very general sense that the dawning of human consciousness seems to have been accompanied, probably inevitably, by a sense of alienation. The geneticist Dobzhansky[2] makes the interesting suggestion that one of the first fruits of self-awareness was the awareness of death, and that it was this contradiction at the heart of life which set humanity on its course. In such speculations there is plenty of scope for exploring the relationship between any empirical claims theologians might want to make and the available scientific evidence. But none of this touches the really fundamental issues, to which we must now turn.

The main threat posed by Darwinism was that it began to close the gaps in the only large remaining area of mystery left to nineteenth-century thought. In a world which seemed to be a vast mechanism pointing only distantly to God as its creator, life, and in particular human life, was a standing witness to God's intimate concern with the details of nature; it was the sphere in which his operations were most evident; it illustrated modes of being beyond the merely mechanistic; and the gulf between animals and humans was the apparently indispensable basis for the Christian doctrine of man. Darwin's ideas challenged all this. Furthermore, they cut at the root of what was then regarded as the most compelling argument for God's existence – the argument from design. Paley's

2. T. Dobzhansky, *The Biology of Ultimate Concern*, 1969.

famous illustration of the watch which demanded the existence of a watchmaker, began to look very different when the
marvellous adaptations of living organisms were seen to
belong only to a tiny, select and successful minority. Organisms adapt because only the adaptable survive.

The issues were central to any theology of God and nature.
We are apt to scoff nowadays at those who base their faith on
a 'god of the gaps', a God whose writ runs only in the remaining areas of human ignorance, and whose territories shrink
as science advances. We see now that there need be no contradiction between scientific and theological interpretations
of the same phenomena, and that theology is concerned with
different questions from science, questions of meaning and
value rather than empirical inter-relationships. It is accepted
that within their own terms, scientific explanations can be
complete and all-inclusive, just as a certain kind of map, as
defined by the purposes for which it was drawn, can tell all
that there is to be known about a particular piece of territory,
without rendering other maps unnecessary. But there are still
many Christians who feel nervous as biologists penetrate more
and more deeply into the intimate processes of life, and who
experience a sense of loss as the story of human development
is unfolded.

Emotionally it is harder for us nowadays to experience the
hand of God in creation because the mystery at the heart of
the universe is rather less obvious than popular religion has
believed. We can illustrate this by returning to the argument
from design. In its legitimate philosophical form this is a
pointer to God which draws out the implications of the fact
that the universe is intelligible to human minds. It ought to
follow from this that the greater the successes of science, the
more compelling the pointer becomes. Paley's version of it,
however, picked on particular instances of design in nature,
and was thus much more immediately appealing. But it col-
lapsed when the particular instances were explained in terms
of a general process.

'The mystery of human life', to give another example,

remains as much of a mystery as it ever was when we think in theological terms about the meaning and purpose of life, the strangeness of existence, the peculiar quality given to our study of life by the fact that we ourselves know it from within, and the unique metaphysical status of the self. All these are unaffected by our understanding of the physico-chemical and developmental sub-structure which underlies our human consciousness, and which may simply add an extra dimension of wonder to our experience. But it cannot be denied that a straightforward scientific mystery is more attractive to many, and that a theology which refuses to appeal to scientific ignorance loses emotionally some of what it gains intellectually.

It follows from this that the character of religion as felt has been profoundly altered by Darwinism, not so much because of any particular biological discoveries, but because the Darwinian controversy more or less completed and brought home to the man in the street the scientific revolution which had begun two centuries before. Although the circumstances of the controversy, the attitudes of church leaders and the personalities involved, must have contributed to this result, the main reason for its enormous impact, of which the echoes are still to be heard, is that for the first time it effectively concentrated scientific attention on the nature of man. Since Darwin the general implications of science for our total understanding of nature, including ourselves, can no longer be ignored.

Apart from this general point, which really requires a treatise on the philosophy of science and religion to do justice to it, there are some special aspects of evolutionary theory which are of theological interest. The shift from a static view of nature to a developing one, for instance, at first seemed to upset the old established order of things. If the world is a process of change, then what sense is it possible to make of such concepts as 'human nature', as if there were some fixed essence of humanity dictating the conditions of our existence. Man is what he has become – and may become. To see man in evolutionary perspective is to realize that countless questions which once appeared to be closed are in fact open. This is undoubtedly threatening, but it is also biblical. The world is not an endlessly repeated series of similar events. Ecclesiastes was quite wrong, as the remaining biblical writers knew he was, in claiming that there was nothing new under the sun. Time, according to the Bible, moves in a significant direction. History might almost be called a device for manufacturing novelty. Far from constituting a challenge to Christian theology, therefore, the evolutionary emphasis on development has revived Biblical insights which were in danger of being neglected. And the view of man which emerges, man as the heir to thousands of millions of years of change, man as a bundle of potentialities rather than a fixed given entity, instead of downgrading him, immeasurably increases his responsibilities.

But what of the human soul? Can this have evolved too? If we think of the soul as some sort of preformed extra faculty implanted by God in the developing human body at a precise moment in time, we face intolerable complications. It is worth noting, though, that these complications are just as great when we consider the embryonic development of a single individual as when considering the evolution of the human race. There is in fact no sharp dividing line between being human and being sub-human, and anybody who has watched the development of a child's personality ought to know this. The whole range of human personal response grows gradually from imperceptible beginnings – including the ability to respond to God. And that surely is what is to be understood by talk about 'the soul'. It is the ability to respond to God; an ability which is partly innate, because it depends for its very possibility on a complex nervous substratum; partly conditioned, because the full range of our responses can only be evoked in a complex social environment; and partly dependent on God himself because we can only respond to one who makes himself known to us. It is in this latter sense that the soul is 'given by God', and it is a sense which does not preclude, but rather demands, an evolutionary account of the soul's origins. It is not for nothing that the world has been called a vale of soul-making. In fact high speculation about God's purposes in creating the world at all would seem to lead to nonsensical conclusions if the most important, enduring and characteristic constituent of human beings could be made by him quite apart from the rest of creation.[3]

Be that as it may, the fact remains that if evolution is God's way of creating, many Christians have had serious reservations about the means. This is perhaps the issue which still causes most trouble to believers who in all other ways are prepared to accept and welcome Darwin's contribution. Even if, as I have suggested earlier, the original picture of 'nature red in tooth and claw' was grossly overdrawn, there is still the nagging problem of a how a process which is essentially and fundamentally based on chance can express the will of a loving Creator.

I believe that the answer to this question, like the only possible Christian answer to the problem of evil, lies in the nature of freedom and of its corollary, creativity. If God's way of creating is to allow the universe to develop through its own inner laws, and thus to exist in relative independence of him, there must be built into the creative process some means whereby this freedom can be generated, and what is genuinely new emerge. I referred earlier to history as a device for manufacturing novelty, which is another somewhat more restricted way of making the same point.

The emergence of novelty has always caused difficulty to philosophers, so much so that some have been tempted to read back into primitive phenomena some minuscule version of the fully developed end-product. Teilhard de Chardin, for instance, fell into this trap when trying to account for the emergence of mind by postulating some fragmentary mind-like attributes extending all the way through nature, right down to the atomic level. But this is an unnecessary and meaningless complication in his system. A new type of motor

3. John Hick in his Eddington Lecture *Biology and the Soul* (1972) has an interesting treatment of this whole subject.

car is not made possible by the presence of potential motor car-like properties in its constituent parts. Newness in such circumstances is essentially new organization or new levels of organization, and creativity is the discovery and exploitation of new combinations or types of combination.

It is possible to illustrate how this happens from the fairly familiar experience of thinking up new ideas. One way of doing this is to allow the mind to play around a subject until out of the blue, as it were, something crops up which seems interesting or suggestive or worth pursuing. Then begins the hard process of thinking out the implications, which may end in the idea being rejected, whereupon the whole business has to start all over again. Sometimes, however, the idea proves fruitful, and the line of thought which stems from it survives. The two essentials in this process are, first the free play of ideas and secondly the selection by trial and error of anything potentially valuable which the play has produced. The word 'play' is significant here. The point is that this is not conscious rational effort, but the deliberate exposure of the mind to what happens to pass through it. And the greater the variety of such thoughts, the greater the chances are that one of them will prove useful. The element of randomness at one stage in the process, throwing up all sorts of hitherto unsuspected possibilities, is precisely what enables the second stage to select and develop ideas which might never have occurred as a mere logical extension of what had been thought of before. Randomness, in other words, can play an important role in creative thinking, without in the least implying that the results of such thinking are 'mere chance'.

The analogy with evolution is obviously not exact. Natural selection is not a conscious agency deciding which new genetic combinations are going to prove fruitful. But neither is it a mere sieve filtering out the weakest and unfittest. The recent developments in evolutionary theory have shown it to be an extremely sophisticated means of testing the implications of such new combinations in a highly complex and changing environment. It is a means, moreover, which especially favours the evolution of intelligence because this in turn increases its sophistication even more. It is not by itself creative, just as chance by itself is not creative. But the conjunction of the two does offer a plausible explanation of how newness emerges, one which has the further advantage of at least resembling our own experience of creativeness.

In a universe which offers vast possibilities of choice, evolution by random variation and natural selection ensures that a wide variety of the possible modes of being should be explored. Teilhard de Chardin appositely used the word 'groping'. 'It means pervading everything so as to try everything, and trying everything so as to find everything.'[4] The profusion of life, the immense variety, the mistakes, the deadends and the failures all make sense on this view of things. Free creativeness drawing on an inexhaustible well of randomness is bound to lead to tragedy and waste and suffering. But it also seems to be the only possible basis for those higher levels of freedom in terms of which Christians have always defended God's wisdom in creation. The alternative, a universe planned in detail and unfolding inexorably as preordained, containing no source of unpredictability within itself, would not only be intolerably dull but also unforgivably evil. Why should whole species be created only to be exterminated? Why should the apparent design of some parts of many organisms be so remarkably inefficient? Why death, unless its counterpart reproduction were essential as a generator of newness?

I wrote earlier that I thought theologians ought gladly and gratefully to accept the full implications of Darwin's ideas. I am not the sort of enthusiast who claims that evolution is the gospel Christianity has always been waiting for. Nevertheless, I hope enough has been said to show that despite the difficulties this is a potentially valuable source of theological insight, and that no real alternative is thinkable, either scientifically or theologically.

4. Teilhard de Chardin, ib., p. 110.

2

DOES GOD THROW DICE?

'Time and chance govern all. . . .' Ecclesiastes 9.11

I have chosen this rather gloomy verse from Ecclesiastes because it is almost the only passage in the Bible where the word 'chance' occurs in anything like its modern sense. Let me use it to highlight one of the differences between the biblical world and our own.

The dominating theme of the Bible is that history is in the hands of God, and therefore what happens in history is significant. Men are going somewhere, and how they go and where they go depends on their responsiveness to the God who is doing things in their midst. Above all, life means something because it is God-given, and God can share it.

In the book of Ecclesiastes this sense of God being at work in history has dropped out. History is just one thing after another. It is an endless series of repetitions going nowhere. So most of what happens is pointless. 'It is all one.' 'Time and chance govern all.' All that remains is some vague sense of God as a moral force.

God – or chance?

Purpose – or pointlessness?

This is the dilemma, as posed in the Bible. But posed, I suspect, with special sharpness in our own day, because so much of our experience seems to lend weight to what Ecclesiastes was writing.

This chapter was originally a Sermon preached in Great St Mary's Church, Cambridge, March 1975.

Here is a quotation from an American scientist – a leading writer on evolution:

Man is the result of a purposeless and materialistic process which did not have him in mind. He was not planned.

And here is another on the same theme, from Jacques Monod's book on *Chance and Necessity*:

Chance alone is at the source of every innovation, of all creation. . . . Pure chance, absolutely free but blind, at the very root of the stupendous edifice of evolution: this central concept of modern biology is no longer one among other possible or even conceivable hypotheses. It is today the sole conceivable hypothesis, the only one compatible with observed and tested fact. . . .

Of course, it is not only biologists who respond like this. The sense of purposelessness, of being caught up in a blind and indifferent process, affects all sorts of people who may know nothing about science, and who are only marginally affected by the sort of vision of the world which hard-line scientists put across. In my part of the world, in North-east England, among a working class culture, the sense of purposelessness, of being at the mercy of chance, is much more likely to spring from social forces, than from scientific reflection. But the end-product is the same. 'Time and chance govern all.' Yet the scientific vision of a world governed by chance typifies, and perhaps to some extent underlies, the sense of hopelessness felt by all sorts of non-scientific people. And this is why I am going to concentrate on it.

This is also why I have used a famous quotation from Einstein as the title of this sermon. 'Does God throw dice?' Einstein was worried by the way physics was developing in the aftermath of the quantum theory. He found it impossible to believe that there was a deep-rooted element of indeterminacy in nature. So his question was really a criticism of quantum theory. But fascinatingly, a question posed in moral, even in religious, terms. Surely the man who believes in a rational universe, a godly universe, cannot allow a major place in it to chance!

Nevertheless the answer to Einstein's question seems to be 'Yes'. And the heart of what I want to say to you this evening is that to accept that 'Yes', to accept that God *does* throw dice, does not destroy rationality or godliness. In fact it opens the way to a valid style of Christian faith and life in a scientific world. It may even help us to see why Ecclesiastes has a legitimate place in the Bible.

Suppose we start by designing an imaginary computer. Everybody knows that computers are stupid and literal-minded. They follow their instructions. They operate according to rigid rules. Some of us can think of people like that.

Now suppose we want a computer with a bit of originality – one which can respond to an unforeseen situation in a creative way. How can it be done? By feeding into it a new range of possible responses, and allowing the ordinary computer mechanisms to select the most appropriate one according to whatever rules it is operating by. But how do we know what new possibilities to feed in? The answer is that we don't, if we are facing unknown situations. Therefore the best way of securing the maximum range of response is to feed in new possibilities at random – and the more the better. In other words, randomness channelled through a mechanism which develops and selects what is fed into it, can produce genuine novelty, a creatively appropriate response.

I am told that in the early days when this was done in computers, the random element was provided by a thing called the Generator of Diversity – until somebody tried abbreviating it to GOD.

What I have been describing for computers is parallelled in the process of biological evolution. Random mutation in the genetic material throwing up new possibilities for biological existence, appropriate combinations selected out, first of all in the processes of embryonic development, and then if successful, tested in the actual business of living through many generations – this is the combination of chance and selection which drives the engine of biological creativity. Perhaps in other aspects of the universe as well, it is the element of chance which makes new developments possible. 'Time and chance govern all. . . .'

Is this a godless vision? I do not believe so. I believe we can be misled by phrases like 'blind chance' and 'unplanned development' into thinking that the universe just goes crazily on its way with no God to care or control, and no purpose to be discerned. It is not chance *alone*, or natural selection *alone*, or any rigid law of development *alone*, which allow this creativity. It is all these elements operating together in the kind of world we actually have. An element of freedom, an element of stability, and the demands of appropriateness. What results, therefore, is not just anything. Admittedly the vast profusion of animal life points to the enormous effectiveness of this means of exploring all possible ways of living on earth. But this is not mere randomness. The process produces certain kinds of end product. Just because there is so much competition, just because the environment changes in unpredictable ways, just because the stuff of the world is what it is, there is a pressure to make animal life more adaptable, more flexible, more responsive. I am not so silly as to say that, biologically speaking, if human beings had not evolved somebody ought to have invented us. What I am saying is that this is the kind of world in which human development makes sense. It is not mere accident. No doubt the actual form we have as human beings depends to a large extent on the accidents of evolutionary history – and this is what those who draw pictures of other kinds of intelligent life – little green men on Mars – are implying. But the fact that our world has developed conscious creatures, marvellously responsive creatures, creatures capable of responding to each other and to God, is not, I believe, a mere matter of chance. Nor do I believe that the scientific account of nature requires us to hold that it is.

It is not, therefore, empty talk, to say that this is God's world in which God's purposes are fulfilled. But sometimes Christians have felt it necessary to defend themselves against the full impact of scientific understanding. A month ago the biography was published of one of the greatest and most eloquent men ever to preach regularly from this pulpit – Charles Raven. He taught a whole generation of Christians in this place to welcome the scientific vision of the world. But even he sidestepped the things which the real hard-liners were saying. Chance, as providing the possibility of freedom and creativity; chance, as a component in God's design – these in the last resort he was unwilling to accept. Yet why not?

It seems to me that there can be an immensely exciting vision of a world which God allows real freedom to create itself. It is a vision which can include the scientific picture, and point beyond it. Human beings have real responsibility. We live in a world where all sorts of tragedies occur, where much seems meaningless and cruel. Yet the very openness and unpredictability of nature, which allow these things to happen, provide the raw material of human freedom, human development, and ultimately human love.

Yet this is not the whole story. 'The created universe', wrote St Paul, 'waits with eager expectation for God's sons to be revealed . . . up to the present the whole created universe groans in all its parts as if in the pangs of childbirth.' This is not a scientific account. This is what happens when you look at the whole process the other way round, starting from Christ. The basic Christian claim is that by taking Christ as the clue to what God is doing in the world, we begin to see a purpose even in what seems like senseless waste and tragedy. The process we are involved in must be capable of going somewhere. This must be a world in the making, a world in which history matters, a world where the freedom given us is to be used – and used not just for ourselves but, in St Paul's words, so that the whole universe can 'enter upon the liberty and splendour of the children of God'.

Do the visions meet – the scientific and the Christian? I

believe they do. And a life-style flows from their meeting which we are only very slowly and painfully beginning to learn. Humble freedom. Accepting our responsibility for the natural world. Yet conscious of the way in which we can spoil and exploit and destroy it unless in a deeper sense we have been made free by God.

Let me end with a practical example which has recently become rather topical. Last week a book was published on the use of animals in scientific experiments. It is not an anti-vivisectionist tract, but a sober, factual account of the sort of things which lie behind the statistics of five million experiments performed on animals in this country per annum.[1] It turns out that only a third of these experiments can properly be classed as medical research. A substantial proportion of the remainder are done for purely commercial purposes. Every new cosmetic or toiletry, for instance, of which there are hundreds a year, is tested for toxicity by being stuffed down the throats of a variety of animals: rats, rabbits, dogs – even apes, until half of them die. What sort of a civilization are we, I wonder, which finds it necessary to kill millions of our fellow creatures by feeding them on face creams, floor polishes, bubble bath liquids, lavatory cleansers and anti-freeze additives?

Humble freedom. This is only one tiny illustration of the need to get our perspective right. We are part of nature, yet responsible for it before God. We have the power to refuse the kind of fatalism which says that commercial pressures or so-called scientific necessity must inevitably have the last word. We can deny the pessimism of Ecclesiastes. 'Time and chance govern all.' For surely the writer got it wrong. Time and chance may be the basis of all, they may be the matrix out of which life flows. But the one who governs all is God, who calls us to respond out of the freedom he has given us, and humbly build up the kingdom of God's love.

1. An official breakdown of the figures, published only in 1978, presents a less alarming picture. Some of the experiments are, nonetheless, distasteful.

3

TRUTH AND DR STEINER

If curiosity kills the cat, the cat will at least have the satisfaction of knowing that it dies in a noble cause. Maybe that
is an unfair summary of Dr George Steiner's recent Bronowski
Memorial Lecture[1]. But it is not all that unfair, so let me give
it in his own words:

> Truth matters more than man. . . . It is more interesting
> than he, even when, perhaps especially when, it puts in
> question his own survival. I believe that the truth does
> have a future. Whether we do is less certain. But man alone
> can suppose this. And it is this supposition, first put for-
> ward in the Mediterranean world some 3,000 years ago,
> which is the mark of his glory.

The dominating image in this extraordinary lecture was
the story of Thales, the mathematical wizard, whose mind
was so fixed on the glories of abstract truth that he stumbled
and fell down a well; the archetype of those who put truth
above personal survival; truth which Dr Steiner goes on to
say may contain more subtle threats than causing accidents
to absent-minded professors.

I, too, want to begin with a story, this time a fictional one
told by Ronald Knox. He called it 'The New Sin', and it
began with a small advertisement in the London papers. A
mysterious professor claimed to have discovered a new and

1. Published in *The Listener*, 12th January, 1978.
This chapter was originally broadcast on B.B.C. Radio 3, and published
in *The Listener*, May 1978.

entirely original sin, and had booked the Royal Albert Hall to lecture on it. Speculation was intense. Letters, sermons, articles poured in. Liberal theologians wrote learned essays doubting whether the concept of sin still had meaning. Several of the more daring of the avantgarde claimed to have known all about the new sin for years, and to have committed it frequently. A Jesuit argued that newness in sin was a logical impossibility, in view of the fact that sin was essentially derivative. A member of Parliament drafted a private member's bill banning the new sin, before it was known what it was. But the main fury and frustration was that no seats in the Royal Albert Hall were bookable in advance. Even the newspaper correspondents had to join an immense queue days before the lecture.

When, at last, the moment came and the professor faced his audience, he began by asserting the genuineness of his discovery. And then he turned on them in disappointment. He had expected, he said, to find people fit to receive a discovery of this magnitude, people who appreciated some of the finer points of sin, people who would know how to use the knowledge given them. Instead, all he saw in front of him was the age-old, squalid, sensation-seeking sin of curiosity. And with that, he vanished in a clap of thunder. Ronald Knox adds a footnote: 'And you, dear reader, weren't you curious too?'

Now I do not pretend that the curiosity Knox condemned is in the same league as the noble pursuit of truth, truth at any cost, which Dr Steiner was holding up for our admiration. I simply use this story as a reminder that there is another aspect to this pursuit, an ignoble one; and it is not always clear what aspect we are operating with. Nor is it as clear to me, as it appears to be to Dr Steiner, that the notion of truth is adequately expressed in his ideal of pure, abstract, disinterested knowledge, so far removed from human interests and passions that falling down a well is trivial in comparison.

My first worry about the relationship between the pursuit of truth and vulgar curiosity has a personal aspect to it. When

I gave up a scientific career, 25 years ago, one of the negative
reasons was my inability to answer the question, 'Why?'. Why
spend a life doing research? And the only answer I could then
give, and the answer given by all my colleagues to whom I
put the question, was: curiosity. And somehow, at that stage,
the answer did not seem enough.

I believe in the pursuit of truth, believe passionately in it.
I am convinced that science cannot afford to do without the
notion of truth, unfashionable though it is in some scientific
circles. I dimly see how, in the notion of truth, science and
theology find a valid meeting-point. But I have also learnt
that these are distant ideal and that day-to-day, run-of-the-
mill science is powered by less exotic fuels, of which curiosity
is one. Lower down the scale are ambition, competitiveness,
economic exploitation. The PhD industry and the publica-
tions race are among the sludge at the bottom.

I say this with no intention of being disparaging. To realize
that a whole variety of motives contribute to the total scientific
enterprise does not in the least invalidate the ideals of the
pioneers at the top. Saints are no less saints because they are
part of a church full of sinners. Indeed, their saintliness makes
them even more aware of their own ambiguity and that of the
institution they serve. The pursuit of truth is no less noble an
ideal because those who undertake it have to produce enough
results to finance their research. But a reminder that we are
dealing, not with a simple, isolated ideal, but with a spectrum
of attitudes and a mixture of motives, can at least sharpen
the question: how do we recognize the pure pursuit of truth
when we see it? How can we avoid giving *carte blanche* to
everything which masquerades under the name of science
without destroying the integrity and the creative impulse of
research at its best? It is a question of discrimination.

But therein lies the difficulty. Proponents of 'truth at any
cost', 'publish and be damned', rightly point out that the
higher flights of science have to be sustained by a vast quantity of research of all kinds, whose consequences can only be
known long after it has actually been done. Advocates of

social responsibility in science rightly assert that the pursuit of truth is not such an absolute and overriding value that all other values must be subordinate to it. My own interests have been in the field of medical research, where it is well recognized that there are limits to what can be done to human beings in the pursuit of medical knowledge. To take an extreme example: if it is possible to make a clear discrimination against the Nazi experiments in concentration camps, why is it so shocking to suggest discrimination in other contexts as well?

The discussion is sometimes polarized as if total freedom and dull-witted suppression were the only alternatives. But, in most human affairs, people manage to find a reasonable balance. And the first main point I want to underline is that science is a human affair like any other, and is, therefore, a mixture of good and bad, wisdom and stupidity, idealism and self-seeking, and is falsified if it is blown up and identified without qualification with the main quest of the human spirit. It is a human activity over which human beings ought to learn how to exercise reasonable control.

The comprehensive quest for truth, I would argue, is larger than science. And this pinpoints my second main worry about Dr Steiner's lecture. He recognizes, of course, that the abstract, disinterested, mathematical kind of truth he is commending has its critics. These are dismissed in a few slashing words as 'the drop-outs of reason', a label which may have surprised honest practitioners in other academic disciplines, whose criteria do not match Dr Steiner's for purity. Does truth belong only to the abstruse heights of speculative thought?

In all this there is a disastrous narrowness. Even within the limited field of the philosophy of science, there is a failure to acknowledge what has been happening. Dr Steiner is right to believe that the Greek ideal of contemplative knowledge is under pressure, but not, as he suggests, from a miscellaneous band of drop-outs with a vested interest in social welfare. The pressure has come from scientists themselves, who, because of internal developments within their science, have become less and less inclined to make ultimate truth claims. Theoretical constructions now tend to be vindicated on the grounds that they work. The distinctive feature of modern science, we are told, is successful prediction. Its distinctive value lies in the power which it confers to manipulate and exploit.

This is not to say that the qualities of abstract truth-seeking – disinterested honesty, fearlessness, and so on – have no relevance. On the contrary, in the actual practice of science, they are as important as they have always been. But the concept of what is being sought is different. And this difference may have major repercussions on the relationship between the scientific quest and other human ends. If scientific knowledge is essentially the power to manipulate, and is no longer consciously defended in old-fashioned terms as the quest for truth for its own sake, then there is likely to develop a bias within the scientific establishment towards the actual use of that power. Instead of the attempt to know all things possible, the emphasis shifts to doing all things possible. In contrast to Kant's dictum, 'ought implies can', it comes to be assumed that 'can implies ought'. If we can, for instance, change our genetic inheritance, the likelihood is that someone will.

I said earlier that I do not believe science can afford to be without the notion of some ultimate truth to which it is approximating, any more than I believe theology can afford to be without it. But I suggest that the way to do this is not by reasserting some abstract ideal, but by taking seriously what is happening at the opposite pole of knowledge, in history and the humanities. Perhaps what empiricism needs is an injection of the concrete and the personal.

Here I want to shelter behind an immense work of German scholarship, Wolfhart Pannenberg's *Theology and the Philosophy of Science*. In what he calls compositely 'the human sciences', there are basic problems about how to make sense of writings, beliefs, experiences, and institutions different from our own, and perhaps separated from us by great distances in time and space and culture. Biblical scholars were among the first to highlight the issues, because they wanted to know how the religious insights of an ancient culture can be understood in terms valid for today. Their aim was practical. Honest preaching depends on honest biblical interpretation. But the methods developed have a much wider application. It began to be seen that other people's experiences in different cultures can only be understood from within, by critical sympathy, by a slow approximation of viewpoints, a merging of horizons, until communication takes place across the gap.

The general problem is to explore the transmission of meaning. And one of the fascinating conclusions is that meaning itself seems to have a limitless horizon. We never really exhaust the meaning of an event. It is always possible to move outwards from a particular experience of meaning into a larger and larger semantic context, which eventually has to include the future as well. The movement of thought, in other words, is in precisely the opposite direction from Dr Steiner's narrowing and abstraction.

As a Christian believer, I suppose I have a vested interest in talking about meaning in this vast context, because it is one of the levels at which statements about God make sense. My immediate purpose, though, is to make a general point about the interpretation of human activity. It is the study of meaning. And to grasp meaning requires sympathy, a fusion of interest and disinterest, openness and criticism, participation and detachment. The aim, if it is to be successful, must be understanding, not manipulation. The study of unfamiliar cultures is a kind of communication, part of whose effect is on those who are doing the studying. And though it is possible to study other people in order to exploit them, there is an element of conscious dishonesty at the heart of such exploitation, which is not so apparent when it is done to the non-human world of nature.

What I am suggesting is that, just at the time when the hard empirical sciences are finding it difficult to be sure that, in some ultimate sense, they really are exploring the funda-

mental structure of the world, the human sciences are remind-
ing us that the aim is understanding, not power. For them,
the search for truth entails a respect for the objects of study.
Disinterestedness and abstraction are not the whole story.
Knowing includes participating. It requires a true relationship between knower and known. Indeed, one of the interesting questions today is how far this kind of insight can feed
back into the natural sciences, and help to mitigate their
apparent lack of concern with human value.

Let me illustrate this from one of Dr Steiner's own examples. He asks whether genetic inquiry should go forward,
'whatever the social, the human consequence', and picks up
echoes of the notorious dispute over how far ethnic factors,
and in particular the difference between black and white,
affect the inheritance of intelligence. Suppose that, as a result
of rigorous research, he says, it were to become clear that the
genetic factors in intelligence greatly outweigh the environmental factors, what then? Suppose we discover that truth is
incompatible with social justice? Suppose truth is ultimately
inimical to man?

I ask in return: what kind of rigorous research could possibly establish conclusions such as these? Even the seemingly
pure scientific aspects of the questions create problems. The
relationship between heredity and environment is not like the
relationship between two objects, salt and water, in which we
can specify the quantity of one over against the quantity of
the other. Nor is it like the relationship between two processes,
addition and multiplication, which we can apply successively
with greater or smaller numbers. It has a unique historical
dimension to it. It is the story of an interaction, and one of
the elements in the interaction has itself an historical dimension. The environment is what it has become. And how and
why it has become what it is, and how it is experienced and
interpreted by those who belong to it – what it means to them
– is part of its effect.

That is not to say that questions about heredity and
environment, insofar as they apply to human beings, are

insoluble in scientific terms. But it *is* to claim that they cannot finally be detached from the non-abstract, human, participatory end of the scientific spectrum, where values count.

If this is true of seemingly scientific questions, it is even more true of a question like, 'Is truth ultimately inimical to man?' On the face of it, we do not need scientists to pose the question for us. It is posed already by death. The truth that every man must die is about as firmly established, and as inimical to man, as any truth could be. Yet, noble-minded despair is not the only response to it. Men react differently to death, not because they differ about the plain empirical facts, but because they see through them to different levels of meaning. As a Christian, I can scarcely be unaware of death, because a death lies at the heart of my faith, a death in which the ultimate threat becomes the ultimate promise. So, when Dr Steiner sets truth against man, and asks whether man has a future, I answer: 'Thank God, yes.'

4

COMPUTERIZED VALUES

I was told recently about a supermarket in Colorado with computer terminals where customers can test their values. Not all their values, of course. The project, as I heard about it, was mainly concerned with road planning – how to choose the most acceptable route through an area of scenic beauty. The terminals display pictures and diagrams of possible routes, and customers state their preferences. The machine does a quick analysis, and back on the screen comes an assessment of the values expressed in the choice. 'Did I really score nothing for safety, three for beauty, and ten for speed?' says a horrified customer. He readjusts his scale of values and tries again. Gradually, by trial and error, a decision emerges, a decision whose value-content has been separately analysed and understood and acknowledged. Meanwhile back at base a central computer records it all for the benefit of those who actually have to make the final choice.

It is a bit disappointing to have to admit that, when I last heard about it, this particular route still remained unplanned. Is the whole thing then just a useless piece of American gadgetry? Or worse, is it all a monstrous confusion, a muddled attempt to treat values as if they were numbers, and hence to stop them escaping through the meshes of the scientific net? My own first reaction was highly sceptical.

But if, for the sake of argument, we adopt a subjective interpretation of values, if we treat them as generalized pref-

A rejected radio script on *The Biological Origins of Human Values* by G. E. Pugh (R.K.P. 1978). The B.B.C. pundits did not share my enthusiasm for the book.

erences, there seems no inherent reason why we should not try to scale them, and then feed them in at appropriate points in some process of calculation.

This, at any rate, is what is done, and done with great success, in the latest types of value-based decision systems. Let us leave Colorado, therefore, which may seem slightly off-beat, and come to Dr Pugh. Dr Pugh is the President of Decision-Science Applications, and the author of a book which, in my view, could set much traditional thinking about values in an entirely new context. *The Biological Origin of Human Values* is an ambitious book; it ranges from computer science and brain physiology to zoology, anthropology and ethics. But the key to it, the key which gives access to a long series of new insights, is Dr Pugh's practical experience of designing computer systems which incorporate values into their decision-making process.

Take school bussing plans in the United States, for instance. These were worked out by computer for forty urban areas in the late 1960s. It was soon found that if sensible plans were to be produced, then a wide range of objectives and preferences had to be fed into the computer. It was not enough to specify maximum desegregation or an upper limit to journey times. The computer could satisfy both criteria with plans which were obviously absurd in terms of the amount of bussing needed or the inconvenience to individual children. Feed in more preferences, like short journeys, minimum numbers of children bussed, fairness as between different children, and the computer began to produce plans which looked not only practical but intelligent.

The values concerned were simple ones, and easily specifiable. Their numerical equivalents had to be found by trial and error, as in the Colorado supermarket. But the principle of bringing together facts and values in a single numerically based process of decision-making seems established. Whatever the philosophers may say, it works.

It only works, however, if all the relevant values are specified. Omit one, or take the easy way out by assigning zero or infinity to particular values too readily, and the resulting decision may be absurd. In practice it seems that the most sensible decisions are made when the value pattern is complex. This may be why earlier and cruder attempts to relate facts and values within a single process, or to reduce decisions to the terms of a single value, like money, have often been such dismal failures. Complex value systems provide a sort of buffer against the literalmindedness of machine intelligence. And there is even better performance when values are allowed to change appropriately with time. The right preferences at one stage in a process may be quite wrong at another stage, just as in human beings the dominant values may differ with age.

How are facts and values related in a decision system? Dr Pugh lists five essential components, components which he then goes on to compare with their equivalents in the human brain:

First, a data collection procedure, a sensory input.

Secondly, a model of relationships in the environment which defines action alternatives and their consequences. This is our picture of reality. It is a component which, in crude attempts to relate values to actions, has often been overlooked. It is crucial, however, and as the argument develops we see how the need for it provides a basis for the intellectual values. To have an inadequate model of the environment is to act ineffectively.

The third component of a decision system must be a procedure for exploring available action alternatives and estimating their consequences. This is the function of rational thought and imagination.

Fourthly, there must be a method for assigning values to the estimated consequences. In human terms, according to Dr Pugh, this is the fruit of our evolutionary history. What evolution has done is to build into us a complex pattern of primary values, which are simply there inside us as a given datum of experience, and to which all our conscious values, the subject of rational reflection, ultimately relate.

Fifthly and lastly, there has to be a decision mechanism for selecting alternatives that show the best value. We weigh up the consequences, we decide, and we act.

And all these, he says, can happen as well in machines as in men.

From here the argument takes off, and I will not pursue it much further. The brain, we are told, is not merely like a computer; it is a computer. Indeed we are given convincing illustrations of the tricks and dodges built into its mode of functioning in order to economize on its computing capacity. True, the ultimate mystery of consciousness remains, but the role assigned to consciousness fits into the general pattern. It is an aspect of the brain's power of model building; it has evolved through the need for specific, and non-routine, reference to an unpredictable environment. The changing model is the bit we concentrate on.

But more central for Dr Pugh, and more important for my immediate purpose, is the claim that below the level of consciousness are the built-in values which have evolved as an integral part of the human decision system. To accept this is far from making ethics non-rational. As in a computer, there is a secondary system of values, a series of rules of thumb, which have their ultimate roots in the primary values, but which are open to rational reflection and change in the light of changing circumstances. But just as a machine can have a basic programme which is part of its design, and is thus unalterable, so can human beings. We are what evolution has made us.

Put like this there is nothing very novel in Dr Pugh's thesis. The sociobiologists are saying the same sort of thing, and others before them. The study of the evolution of human behaviour has accumulated an enormous literature. The beauty of this particular account, though, is that it provides a consistent model of what behaviour is, and how values function within it. In so doing it bypasses familiar philosophical problems about deriving values from facts. The facts are that values are built into us, and as the argument develops we begin to see how, albeit in a very crude and elementary way, such a system might work. Furthermore the values are not necessarily coherent and compatible; indeed for some purposes it is a positive advantage if they are not. Neither are they merely selfish and animal. The evolution of social and intellectual values is still a matter of speculation and controversy, but in principle it is possible to see how these might fit into the general picture. A successful decision-making system needs to place a high value on co-operation and truthfulness. But one of the inherent difficulties created by evolved value systems is that when social evolution progressively takes over from genetic evolution, the basic programming may be inadequate to cope with radically changing circumstances.

I have spoken at some length about this book because I think it raises many questions for theologians, which are going to need careful answers. The author is not a religious believer, but he goes out of his way to make the point that his thesis is compatible with religious faith. If we are computers, which is what he claims our brains must be, then what is unique about us is not our mode of operation, but the dimensions of reality with which we can make contact. We have been led through history, through experience, through the network of relationships in which we live, through (as I would put it) the leading hand of God, to build up a model of the environment that includes transcendence. The reflection of this in us, insofar as we view ourselves in these computerized terms, is a kind of open-endedness, an aspiration, a spiritual search which lifts us way beyond our origins. Let me put it in more familiar religious language. 'God has made us for himself, and our hearts are restless until they find rest in him.' As against St Augustine's insight the language of computer science may seem barbaric, but there is nothing in it which need be a basic threat to human personality.

The really interesting questions, as I see them, are the ethical ones, because it is on these that a great deal of work in this field is converging. Have we here a new basis for natural law? I am not now referring to scientific laws, but to the ancient ethical tradition that there is somehow built into human nature a set of principles which ought to be discernible by reason. The Christian *locus classicus* is St Paul's reference in the Epistle to the Romans, to the Gentiles who have 'the law of God written in their hearts'. The difficulty about this concept, though, has always been to give it any firm content. It has either been interpreted in highly abstract and generalized terms which have not been of much practical use, or it has been rooted in superficial observations of human nature, which then by a sudden jump in logic become the source of prescriptions about what we ought to do. Popular books on human behaviour and its animal ancestry often make this mistake. But it is inherent, too, in much more subtle discussions of natural law; the most notorious is the anti-contraception argument based on biological statements about the procreative function of sex. A straight-line argument from biology to ethics is suspect, unless somehow within the biology values are being authoritatively expressed. And this is precisely what Dr Pugh claims to give us. The values are there, not in superficial biological structures, not in observable habits which human beings share in common with other animals, but in the innate programming of the human decision system.

There are those who would argue on Christian grounds that all such talk is dangerous, because human nature is fallen. Be our programming what it may, this is no guide to true ethical standards, which are found only in God's revelation. The whole point and promise of the Christian life is to escape the entanglements of the past, including our evolutionary entanglements; and to accept what evolution has made us as a guide to what we must be, would be sheer apostasy.

I accept the force of this objection. In its sharpest form it is an objection against natural law as such. But in its more defensible forms I believe it is a warning to be careful, not to set limits to what human beings can become by concentrating on their starting point rather than on their destiny. An understanding of human nature, an understanding such as I have tried to develop, which allows a central place to the response to the transcendent, maybe can escape this danger. Again let me put it in more familiar religious terms: The law written in our hearts can become the law of Christ in those whose hearts are open to him. The natural man is not destroyed but redeemed. The innate imperatives are not over-ridden, but find new levels of fulfilment.

Despite the dangers and limitations, the search for some new formulations of natural law is important, if only as common ground on which religious believers and others can begin to tackle some of the ethical problems of our day. Digging out and exposing innate human values, even if they exist in identifiable forms at all, is not going to be easy. The very idea has already encountered fierce opposition on political grounds from those who place their hopes for mankind on social conditioning. There are enormous difficulties, both practical and theoretical, in trying to separate out the different components in anything as complex and as fluid as human behaviour. But it nevertheless seems to me overwhelmingly probable that some innate values are sufficiently powerful and sufficiently stable to act as fixed points around which the search can go on. How strongly they determine our behaviour, how amenable they are to change, and how we can be sure when we have found them, have all still to be discovered. And it could be that when the answers to some of these questions are known, the insights of novelists and poets and prophets and saints will still go on telling us much more about human nature than the carefully distilled conclusions of sociobiologists or experts in computers.

Nevertheless, I hope the search will go on, and that out of it, and perhaps out of other disciplines as well, a new and better based natural law will develop. Our human consciousness that there are norms and criteria which we disregard at our peril, needs to be strengthened. There is a wisdom in nature, a wisdom which may find some difficulty in adjusting itself to our sophisticated world; but we are the better for knowing it.

5

SCIENCE AND MORAL EDUCATION

To deliver the Macmillan Education Lecture must surely be accounted as a privilege to those who are professionals in the field of education; how much more to one who is decidedly amateur! I am not an educationalist. It is twenty years since I last taught science, and then only at University level. My approach, therefore, is that of an outsider, one who has a broad interest in scientific education but little remaining expertise, and who is probably dreadfully out of date.

Yet I have a personal interest in the subject, because it was the experience of teaching science which made me aware of the many other and more human problems, which gave my students greater trouble than the relatively simple technical matters I was paid to elucidate for them. And this was the beginning of a way of thinking which led me eventually to my present job. In those days science and moral education, and – even more – religious education, seemed poles apart. Nowadays, I hope and believe this is not so. Indeed my main objective is to demonstrate that science has a vital role in moral education, and is itself better taught through being brought into relationship with this broader human context.

By 'science' I mean the natural sciences, the traditional school subjects. The moral significance of disciplines like psychology and the social sciences is obvious, and anything I say about the natural sciences applies even more forcibly to them. But I assume that in the context of school science they are not relevant.

This chapter was the Macmillan Education Lecture delivered to the Association for Science Education, Jan. 1975.

The phrase 'moral education' needs more explanation, and I take as a convenient starting point a recent debate which took place on the subject in the House of Lords. The object of the debate was to draw attention to the work of the Social Morality Council which, in the few years of its existence, has done much to foster the idea of moral education as something distinct and separable from religious education. Council members include Christians, Humanists, Jews, and Muslims, and they are committed to search together for fundamental values which can unite them despite their differences of religious belief. Their avowed object is 'to promote morality in all aspects of the community'.

It was pointed out in the debate that there are many other bodies concerned with moral education in this broad sense, notably the schools themselves. But probably the most convenient and authoritative summary of current thinking is still the Council's Report on *Moral and Religious Education in County Schools*, published in 1970. 'Moral education', it says, 'is the business of everybody in the school and not merely of the head or the R. E. staff. It is not a subject in the timetable, but an aspect of everything that is taught and everything that is done in the school, including not least the way in which the school is organized and run.' Later on in the report, and of more particular concern in the present context, it is recommended

> that every boy and girl should leave school with some understanding of the 'human programme', the global tasks and problems and possibilities which face mankind today and bind us together as human beings living under the same threats and promises which spring mainly from the new and growing powers of a world-wide scientific culture. A young person needs a perspective on his responsibility to share in the care and improvement of his world.

It might seem from this as if the very broad scope of moral education must obviously include science as one of its central concerns. Indeed, as long ago as 1957 The Science Masters' Association said as much in their Policy Statement *Science and Education*:

> Science must be recognized and taught as a major human activity which explores human experience and then maps it, methodically but also imaginatively, so as to make coherent, reliable and communicable sense of it. . . . Each science or group of sciences is concerned only with a limited aspect of human experience abstracted from the whole. As a human quest for Truth – and it is much more subjectively human than is generally realized – science is concerned with one of the main values and qualifies for the status of an active humanity. The schools, therefore, have the duty of presenting science as part of our common and human-istic heritage; it should be taught in harmony with, not in opposition to, the various Arts subjects which alone have hitherto been regarded as humanities.

I do not know how far this policy has actually been carried out, but it has clearly not penetrated far in Governmental circles. In replying to the debate on the Social Morality Council, to which I have referred, the Government spokesman, Lord Melchett, said: 'So far as the actual curriculum is concerned, I doubt whether it is possible to study, say, English or history, without being involved in the consideration of . . . social and moral questions.' No mention of science. Indeed, I cannot recall even the most indirect reference to it in two hours of debate. On the principle that people reveal more about their real thinking by what they inadvertently omit than in thought-out policy statements, it seems that at least in some circles science and moral education are not considered to have much to do with one another.

Before suggesting some reasons why this may be so, let me make a personal interjection. I have referred to the work of the Social Morality Council, for which I have deep admiration and sympathy. I believe that in the present pluralist state of our society, where religious agreement is hard to find, the attempt to detach moral education from its traditional religious basis is important and should be encouraged. But I do not believe that, in the end of the day, it can wholly succeed. Our moral outlook must depend in the last resort on our total views of the world and man and human destiny, and these in turn depend on beliefs, or the absence of beliefs, about God. It is not a question of religiously authoritative moral codes, but of ultimately inescapable questions about the sort of creatures human beings are. And these are religious questions.

I have deliberately used the phrases 'in the end', 'in the last resort', 'ultimately', because before reaching 'the last resort' there is plenty of intermediate ground where useful things can be said and done without raising divisive religious issues; and it is on this intermediate ground that the Social Morality Council stands, and where I stand in this lecture.

But now, having indicated where, in my view, religious commitment fits into the picture, I must return to my main theme. Why do some people regard science as having a less prominent part to play in moral education than other disciplines?

A preliminary set of difficulties centres around the word 'authority'. I hope nobody these days is still wedded to the crude contrast between an authoritarian ethics and the open-minded scientific search for truth. Some religious moral pronouncements may still seem to give substance to it, and no doubt some scientists have still not absorbed the lessons philosophers and historians of science have been teaching them about the, at times unreasonable, and even obscurantist, tenacity of scientific commitments. But by and large it is increasingly accepted that both morally and scientifically we have to learn by initiation into a tradition, and this entails respect for and acceptance of authority. The *Durham Report*[1] put it thus:

---

1. *The fourth R. The Durham Report on Religious Education*, paras. 157-8.

The student of religion or morality, the student of science or history, needs to be inducted into the tradition of these disciplines, a process which involves both learning how to think in the appropriate ways and accepting a good deal on authority. An education in any of these fields would be a failure if it produced people who were subservient and uncritical; it would also be a failure if it produced people who supposed that they could themselves re-write the entire subject from scratch. Hence 'openness' does not require us to proceed as if we were operating in a cultural vacuum – it cannot mean 'not having any presuppositions, not accepting anything which one cannot here and now justify to any reasonable man, not being prepared to accept anything on authority'. Openness must mean 'not being doctrinaire, encouraging people to think for themselves, being ready to consider arguments against one's own position'.

Yet when all this is said, there remains a contrast between moral and scientific education, which cannot wholly be removed by stressing the open element in ethics and the authoritative element in science. Moral demands are some-how inherently authoritative in a way in which scientific statements are not. Ethics is *about* authority. Indeed no less a person than Kant pinpointed the heart of morality precisely here. Moral goodness is the recognition of and response to a claim. We may arrive, as Kant tried to do, at the notion of this claim by rational argument. We must certainly argue about the contents of the claim, and not accept them as merely given. But what makes the claim peculiarly moral is that it has an authority over us; it refers not merely to what we have decided to do or think is rational to do, but to what we ought to do. Morality somehow introduces a different dimension, what Kant called 'duty', and what we might more loosely describe as the sense of values outside ourselves, impinging on us, rather than generated by us.

Kant is not very fashionable these days, but no moral

education worthy of the name should ignore this strand in ethical thinking. Without the sense of over-riding obligation, without the sense that there are imperatives which transcend our situation, morality becomes a poor thing, the reflection of a particular culture, with no power to resist the gradual erosion of values or the encroachments of totalitarianism.

Where such an authoritative approach to morality can go wrong is in becoming prematurely rigid. Over-riding obligations and absolute imperatives are not the sort of things which can be spelt out in day-to-day moral codes. They are more like a receding horizon, a constant reminder of the direction in which we must go, and of our present lack of insight and attainment. Meanwhile all particular appeals to moral authority must be scrutinized and criticized. And this is where moral concern and the scientific spirit can interact fruitfully while respecting each other's differences. There is much to be learnt, I believe, by honest and informed discussion of the role of authority in different aspects of life and of academic study. But this can only be done if the stereotypes of authoritarianism and openness are first disposed of, and we concentrate instead on the ways in which our respective authorities are tested. What is the relationship, for instance, between scientific experiment and moral experiment? I wonder if such a question is ever discussed in the classrooms, and if so what answers emerge.

Closely related to this theme of authority is the distinction between fact and value. I suggest this as a second obstacle discouraging some from making full use of science as part of moral education. Let me introduce the point by quoting from a leading article in *New Scientist*, reporting on the first conference of geneticists and molecular biologists, held to discuss the benefits and hazards of genetic engineering. Main publicity was given to the now famous proposal by Paul Berg for a moratorium on certain types of experiments which might by accident spread antibiotic resistance to important pathogenic bacteria, or disseminate cancer-inducing genes among the human population. Berg explained that his decision had nothing to do with ethics. 'It is simply a public health problem.' When asked what he would do if, as a result of his proposal, his research was no longer wanted, he replied: 'I'd stop it if there was a sound practical reason, but not if it were an ethical judgment.' Whereupon a molecular biologist rushed to support Berg by suggesting that what basic researchers do is unearth facts, 'and facts have no ethical connotation'. 'Anyway', he added, 'ethics change with time'. The leading article commented: 'He would be right, of course, if facts never escaped from their laboratory, but in real life they have a habit of creeping through the door and changing the world. . . .'

I quote this at some length because it is easy to assume that the relationship between fact and value, with all its corollaries for the ethical responsibility of scientists, has now been so thoroughly explored that there is little scope for disagreement. However, when top scientists, at a conference convened to discuss ethical problems, so obviously still feel that their research is not subject to ethical judgements, it is worth questioning the assumption that all is well.

There is always a certain nervousness among scientists about allowing questions of value to affect their work. Science only achieved its successes when all such questions were rigorously exluded. Part of its mythology is that objective facts, and these alone, feed the scientific enterprise, and the intrusion of any other influence, whether political, religious, or moral, produces fatal distortions.

It is well known that in practice the story of scientific progress is not quite so simple, and that scientists as human beings have been just as much involved in value judgements as anybody else, including value judgements that their own work is a proper responsible human activity. It is claimed, however, that none of this human fallibility need affect genuine scientific objectivity, because the processes of communication and testing ensure that in the long run distortions caused by personal factors are ironed out. Science is thus self-correcting, despite the shortcomings and biases of individual scientists, and in this general sense it is possible to claim that it is value-free.

The trouble is that it is individual scientists, and not an entity called 'science', who have to make decisions about what research is done and how it is used. And for individuals the secure sense of being part of a self-correcting process can generate its own temptations. The individual may feel that he can contract out because the process itself will take care of any dangers or evils his work may give rise to. Professor Medawar coined a phrase which expresses perfectly this attitude. 'New skills for new ills.' In other words, don't be alarmed by the apparent implications of some scientific research, because science will always have the capacity to keep one step ahead.

I do not share his optimism, not least because all the evidence goes to show that new ideas and new techniques once released rapidly become uncontrollable. Whereas at an earlier stage in scientific history a new discovery could have a very limited application and a long period of testing, nowadays a new advance may be publicized on a world-wide scale before it is even properly established. The scare over the supposed relationship between XYY chromosomes and criminal tendencies is a case in point. How many people were penalized for having the wrong chromosomes before the inadequacy of the original research was revealed?

Moral awareness and a sense of social responsibility must begin with the individual scientist himself. Therefore it seems to me that those who educate the scientists of the future have an important task to ensure that science is studied within a moral context. Perhaps this is best done, and is no doubt already done, by teaching science as a human activity, a vital part of civilized life, but only a part, which needs constantly to be related to the whole. The study of the lives of individual scientists with all their mistakes and confusions and irrelevancies was sadly neglected in my day. Instead, the impression was conveyed to us by our text books that everything followed with a sort of logical inevitability, correct, passionless, precise. Accounts of scientific discovery which highlight the elements of passion, commitment, and sheer partisanship help us to see some of the moral issues as they have arisen, and how they were faced or avoided.

No doubt the trend towards integrated studies has already brought traditional science partly out of its isolation. The goal I referred to earlier of studying 'global tasks and problems and possibilities' presupposes a multi-disciplinary approach in which moral, political, scientific and technical questions are all inter-related. But it is worth noting in passing what extraordinary strains such integrated teaching must place on the teachers. In studying, say, a problem like world population, it is no easy matter to recognize all the separate strands and to keep the balance between scientific evidence, political expediency, technical feasibility, and moral insight. This is yet another reason, it seems to me, for encouraging the sensitive exploration of the relation between fact and value. Scientists need encouragement and help in accepting their role in moral education, just as those concerned with the humanities must be taught to see science as their ally and to have a proper respect for scientific evidence.

My third suggestion as to why science may hitherto not have played much part in moral education may no longer be applicable. I can approach it through words written by Max Born some 30 years ago. He wrote:

Long years of neglect have not deleted the deep impression made in my youth by the age-old attempts to answer the most urgent questions of the human mind; the questions about the ultimate meaning of existence, about the Universe at large and our part in it, about life and death, truth and error, goodness and vice, God and eternity. But just as deep as this impression of the importance of the problems is the memory of the futility of the endeavour. There seemed to be no steady progress as we find in the special sciences, and like so many others, I turned my back on philosophy and found satisfaction in a restricted field where problems can actually be solved.[2]

The title of an admirable little book by Medawar on the nature of science, called *The Art of the Soluble*, seems to echo the same concern. Science, unlike philosophy, ethics, theology or the humanities in general, tackles problems which can actually be solved. Therein lies its strength – and its temptation.

The temptation, of course, is to imagine that the great human problems, if neglected, cease to be relevant. In a man of Max Born's wisdom and personal stature this may not matter so much; in any case the problems came back to him at the end of his life and gave rise to the essay from which I have quoted. But in an adolescent beginning to specialize in science, and perhaps subconsciously wanting to escape from personal problems which have become too threatening, a morally vacuous and restrictive approach to scientific teaching can be permanently stunting.

I am not sure whether such an escape into science is possible in these days, and this is why what I am saying may not be applicable. But in my own day it certainly was; and a glance at my children's scientific text books suggests that it still might be.

Take an obvious example. The biologist studies plants and animals. Man is treated as part of biology insofar as he is an animal, and since there are usually initial resistances to be overcome against thinking of ourselves merely in these terms, the tendency is to play down any features of man which might seem to be unique. All this may be perfectly correct and scientific. But as part of a total educational programme it can easily become seriously distorting. It can seem on the surface as if students are being taught about the nature of man, whereas the very things which are distinctively human are left out. Sex education, for instance, as a topic in biology, unrelated to teaching about human personality and society

2. The Joule Memorial Lecture, Manchester 1950.

and the poetry of love, may well do more harm than good. Technical factual information, isolated from its human and moral context, may merely serve to depersonalize what ought to be most deeply personal.

Practice obviously varies enormously. But the general point that scientific teaching, unrelated to a wider context, can impoverish a developing personality seems to me to be well established. Near the beginning of Sommerhoff's *Analytical Biology* – an old book now, but an important one in its day – there is a lyricai passage in which he describes the growing sense of wonder in the adolescent learning about the marvellous adaptations and intricacies of the world of nature.

But then [he goes on] arrives the day when he learns how most of these phenomena can be causally accounted for in terms of physics and chemistry, and the hit and miss of natural selection. The romance comes to a sudden end, his original wonder and sense of divine mystery suddenly find themselves opposed by authoritative scientific voices telling him to regard all these phenomena as no more than the chance results of essentially blind physico-chemical forces, and as cosmologically insignificant. From the social and religious point of view a valuable attitude of mind is often lost thereby. Living nature ceases to be something with which man can enter into personal relationships.

Sommerhoff goes on to say that the ability of the adolescent to cope with this kind of discovery must depend to a large extent on the character and temperament of his teachers. If an adolescent is tempted to avoid his human problems by plunging into science as a purely objective study with no concern for moral values, his plight is made even more disastrous if his teachers have done the same.

So far my theme has been a negative one. I have indicated three areas of resistance against fully integrating science into moral education, and I hope that in so doing I have also been able to suggest ways in which the resistances could be overcome, or at least be put to profitable use. I now turn to the positive side of the picture, and conclude by giving two examples of the sort of contribution I believe science can make.

First, and most generally, science is itself a source of values. I have in mind the kind of character training which is necessary to produce a successful scientist. Openness, honesty, a readiness to accept criticism, patience, persistence, a love of truth for its own sake, accuracy, objectivity, co-operativeness and mutual trust – these are all qualities of immense importance in any society, not least our own. To bring these values and attitudes to bear on our moral discussions lifts them on to a new plane of seriousness and relevance. Far too much moralizing goes on in the absence of factual evidence and without the spirit of careful investigation which it is second-nature for a well-trained scientist to bring to any enquiry. The point is an obvious one, but perhaps I can add two footnotes.

One is to draw attention to the interesting way in which values and attitudes, once forming the cultural and religious matrix in which modern science grew, are now often fed back in criticism of that culture. Science has in fact become self-authenticating. The values which supported it have been justified by success. It no longer seems to need external moral vindication. In the extreme form of this doctrine, the progress of science is itself the sole criterion of excellence; what promotes the scientific attitude is good; what denies or stultifies it is bad.

Such a view has dangers, in that a mature culture recognizes a balance, and often a conflict, of values. To make one value, even so fundamental a one as the pursuit of knowledge, supreme over all the others could open the door to a kind of scientific totalitarianism. None of this is meant to detract from what I have said about the importance of scientific values, but it is to emphasize again that science is to be understood as one activity among others in a wider human context.

My other footnote concerns my own experience in recent

years in trying to teach theology to a number of ex-scientists. On the whole I have found them a joy to deal with. They are stimulating because they ask for evidence, where many brought up in other disciplines are content with ideas. And this puts a theologian on his mettle to an unusual degree. But I have also noticed a curious tendency to religious fundamentalism among scientists, and I suspect that this relates to the kind of explanation which they are used to handling in their scientific studies. They look for a clarity, an objectivity and a definiteness which are in fact unobtainable in the murkier and more humanly complex waters of religion and ethics. It is dreadfully easy for scientists to be religiously and morally naive.

So much for my general point about science as a source of values, a fruitful source, but not the sole one. My second example of the kind of positive moral contribution I believe science can make is a personal one drawn from physics. I deliberately refrain from cashing in on present-day concerns about energy policy, pollution, nuclear proliferation, and all the other major questions which scientific advances have posed. Presumably this is a line of teaching which is already thoroughly exploited. For me physics became morally and religiously educative to a unique degree the first time I really understood the kinetic theory of gases. This was a moment of wonder. In fact I believe that it was my first deep religious experience. It was also a moment of humility and delight, as a sense of the orderliness and the givenness of the world first really hit me. Why this particular theory, as opposed to many others, struck me in this way, I cannot now remember, but no doubt it was the way it was taught. The discovery that a mental construction could more or less fit the facts of nature was not presented as yet another example of human ingenuity, but as a revelation to be contemplated, an experience of beauty.

Old-fashioned scientists used to make a great deal of the sense of wonder, and some of the greatest of them still do. Nowadays when considerations of usefulness are paramount, it tends to be a somewhat neglected quality, and I suspect that there has been a corresponding loss of humility. We live in the age of the expert, and experts by definition lack humility.

Yet contemplation is coming back; witness the varied forms adopted by the religious search. And a technological culture desperately needs the counterbalancing quality of humility. Technical competence can breed a certain brashness and arrogance, which become highly dangerous when found in those who wield actual power. The concentration of various kinds of power in relatively few hands in sophisticated technological societies, therefore, makes enormous demands on the quality of their moral education. For these people, often in key positions in our society, much depends on the spirit in which they learnt their science.

Humility before the facts, humility in the face of ignorance, wonder at the splendour and complexity of the whole – these are qualities which even a science far removed from central human concerns can validly evoke. The fact that in the past some thinkers have slid too easily from doing science to 'thinking God's thoughts after him', and have been apt to gloss over the difficulties and inconsistencies too readily, should not, I believe, deter us from trying to teach science in this spirit. A morality which begins with wonder and humility will not go far wrong.

6
BE LIKE GOD

Big conferences tend to drown us in words. But the words which stick, the words which rouse the heart and mind to action, usually have to be rather few and simple. We depend on symbols, images, phrases to carry our meaning. And if what is said inside a conference is ever to penetrate outside it, it is the symbols and images which have to carry most of the weight.

People who know little or nothing of nuclear energy have heard of 'The Faustian bargain'. Many who are only dimly aware of the mixed blessings of scientific curiosity will nevertheless talk of Pandora's Box, though they might be embarrassed if pressed to explain who Pandora was or what her box contained. And it is the same with Prometheus, and perhaps even with lambs and wolves – images, all of them helping to focus debate. More accurate and sophisticated phrases like 'the just participatory and sustainable society' lack force, lack emotional grip, outside the context of the discussion which produces them.

But where are the biblical images in this process? Why do we have to go to Greek mythology? Is it that the biblical writers were basically uninterested in the themes of our Conference? I hardly think so, for they touch the deepest issues in the relationship between God and his creation. Or is it

This chapter was originally a sermon entitled 'Faith, Science and the Future', preached on Sunday, 15 July 1979 at the Ecumenical Service of Worship in Old South Church, Boston, Massachusetts, on the occasion of the World Conference on *Faith, Science and the Future*, organized by the World Council of Churches. The Conference slogan was 'a just, participatory and sustainable society'.

that the biblical imagery has somehow been spoilt, over-played, so that it is difficult to see beyond the interpretation which history has put on it? This is nearer the mark, I suspect. And this is why I ask you in hearing my text to hear it just as it is. I am not now concerned with critical scholarship or with uncritical literalism, but with a story, an image, which lives and grows in the pages of the Bible, and draws into itself the fundamental themes of our Christian faith: the story of the godlikeness of man.

Genesis 3. 1-5: 'Now the serpent was more subtle than any other wild creature the Lord God had made. He said to the woman, "Did God say, 'You shall not eat of any tree of the garden?' " And the woman said to the serpent, "We may eat of the fruit of the trees of the garden: but God said, 'You shall not eat of the fruit of the tree which is in the midst of the garden, neither shall you touch it, lest you die'. " But the serpent said to the woman, "You will not die. For God knows that when you eat it your eyes will be opened, and you will be like God, knowing good and evil." '

The serpent is not some great demonic tempter. We are told simply that he was 'subtle', 'clever'. This is the tempta-tion of cleverness, which sees beyond any arbitrary limits set on human activity, and opens up vistas of knowledge and power which could set man beside God himself. 'You will be like God, knowing good and evil.' There is a striking interpret-ation of the text on one of the murals in the Walter Hall in the Massachusetts Institute of Technology. Instead of a ser-pent there is a white coated scientist dispensing the blessings of knowledge. I don't know whether the artist was being ironic; perhaps he was just drawing attention to the poten-tiality of science for good or evil. But in one respect at least he got it right. The knowledge promised to those who eat the fruit is not just moral insight. 'Good and evil' is a vivid phrase for 'everything'. This then is the promise: you shall know 'everything'. It is the fascination of unlimited knowledge, godlike knowledge, which is man's glory – and his downfall.

In one sense the promise was true – at least in biblical

terms. Humanity, we are told, alone bears the image of God. Humanity, in these old stories, is alone given dominion over the fish of the sea and the birds of the air and over every living thing. Humanity alone shares consciously in God's activity as creator.

But equally, only human beings know that they must die. Only human beings know their separation from God, know the frustrations and limitations of creatureliness. Only human beings can plunge into the abyss of rootless, unrestrained, demonic freedom.

It is a familiar paradox; the same paradox that the Greeks knew only too well. But in the pages of the Bible it gains in depth and power, because it is the first step in a whole series of rich theological themes. One could write most of Christian theology around it. God became man that man might be lifted up to God. But though man is himself made in the image of God, it is his godlike pretensions which lie at the heart of his misery. It is in the resolution of this paradox that salvation lies. But if, on the other side of this paradox, man can indeed become godlike, can indeed share God's knowledge and power, then what have we to learn from God's own use of his power? And if it is true that the image of God in us, even in the best of us, always remains a broken and distorted image, then how dare we impose on God's creation the distortions of our own egotism? A rich and complex theme.

'Who is man?' asked a Jewish writer. 'A being in travail with God's dreams and designs.' But he went on to say, 'how embarrassing to be a messenger who forgot the message.'

Godlike knowledge: a rich theme but a dangerous one. Is the concept so tarnished nowadays, even in science, that we had better abandon it? Human knowledge, we are constantly reminded, is inevitably partial, limited, conditioned. Our concepts, even our scientific concepts, belong to a time and a place and a social setting. The search for truth in some absolute sense is a relic of the religious past and of the scientific age of innocence. The most that any of us can have, we are now told, is a map of things from our own particular point of view and, the severer critics would add, ministering to our own particular advantage.

But isn't this going too far? Aren't we being invited to a treason of the scientists every bit as destructive and dangerous as the treason of the clerics? Science surely is and must be the search for reliable knowledge: a search which can go wrong, which can be corrupted, which is only partially successful, and in which the results are always provisional. But within its limits it actually produces reliable knowledge, knowledge we rely on every day. Within its limits it produces concepts so well tested, and ideas so fundamental, that we are justified in saying, 'This corresponds in some fashion to the way things really are.' Is this dangerously godlike?

To deny it, to deny that there are truths we can at least approximate to, in my view cuts away the ground from religion as well as from science. Indeed, in a curious way science needs the concept of religious truth. It needs a kind of overarching awareness of some ultimate reality, a reality which is what it is, and is not a mere projection of our own inadequacies, a reality to which belief in God bears witness. To me concern for truth and concern for God are two sides of the same coin.

But it is important not to read too much into this. If we human beings are only in some distorted fashion god-like, if we are trapped in our own particular points of view, conditioned by who we are and where we are, then it is not enough just to equate our truth with God – and leave things there. The way to truth, to unity of perception, is much more costly than that. The Gospel is that God doesn't just stand there as some sort of ultimate truth. He enters into our human points of view, and shares them, and slowly bridges the gulfs between them, if we will let him, and offers us the promise of transcending them, and meanwhile bears the pain of our distortions and divisions. We too are not to be godlike spectators searching for patterns in a universe which somehow already reflects the unity of God. We are fellow workers invited, incredibly, to share in the costly work of creating a universe.

We are to 'make sense' of it: 'make' in the active sense, not just in the passive sense.

'You will be like God.' How do we do it? How should we exercise our powers as creators, creators even of new forms of life itself? How should we use and share and develop and respect the resources God has put at our disposal? How far should we work in partnership with things as they are, going along the grain of nature, and how far against it? How far can we correct by fallible human planning the complex system of checks and balances, structures and traditions, which life has evolved?

These are some of the questions we are here to wrestle with. We know perfectly well that there are no general answers. But if we are to respond to them as fellow-workers with God, entrusted with at least some bit of godlikeness however distorted, then perhaps we might find a clue to a right approach in asking how God himself uses his powers, how he interferes, how he works within and against the forces of the world.

'God so loved the world that he gave. . . .' To care is to interfere: but to interfere subtly, in the form of a servant, so that the bruised reed is not broken and the smoking flax not quenched. The character of God's care is that it is incarnated, localized, rooted in the world itself. Perhaps this is where some of our human work reveals its failings.

Let me illustrate. Why are people so suspicious of Trans-national corporations? One reason, I suspect, is that they don't really belong anywhere. They are not rooted, localized, commited to a particular place. And so they can afford to be insensitive to local needs and feelings and values. I am not saying that they must be. But it is part of the price we pay for a mobile society that we become less sensitive to exploitation.

To care is to interfere. But caring must entail local root-edness. Of course, we cannot really go back to our enclosed, isolated, immobile little social systems, where all caring can be direct and personal. Perhaps the way ahead is to learn to

see the world itself as a local place in a universe of immens-
ities. Only one earth: and a shrinking one at that.

God's interference also demands responsiveness. His power
is the power to evoke, not to overwhelm. I once coined the
phrase that 'God acts by being believed in'. It is not wholly
true, but it makes a point. The story of faith in God is, at
least in part, the story of how something new and vital is fed
into the stream of history by those who respond to what they
see as the call and presence of God. It is effective, I believe,
because God is actually calling. But for the moment it is the
element of response I wish to stress. God acts through people
who respond to him. And so to act with truly godlike power
must surely be to evoke responsiveness in others. Is this the
theological basis of participation?

One final point – the point to which any sermon on this
theme must eventually lead. God's action, God's caring,
God's power finds its focus in the cross. This is the heart of
the paradox of godlikeness. This is where human godlikeness
brings God, and where God's humanity finds man. Here is
the place of judgement and hope. And though it is here that
I end, perhaps it is really here that we ought to begin.

The trouble about conferences, as I said at the start, is the
multitude of words: fine words, moving words, intelligent
words, words designed to change the world. But the reality
I suspect we are most conscious of is ignorance and confusion.
We grope our way through monstrously difficult problems,
snatching at insights, carefully balancing our differences. The
bigger the conference, the longer the years of preparation, the
more intense the efforts, the more generous the supplies of
scholarship, the more conscious we are of our ultimate inadequacy. But it is just then, in the failure of our godlikeness,
that we can dare to go to the man on the cross. 'Would you
be like God?' he asks us. 'Then you can attain it only by
sharing the pain and the darkness, the self-giving and the
self-restraint, of God's way of being God.'

PART TWO

THE ETHICAL DIMENSION IN SCIENCE AND TECHNOLOGY

7
THE PROLIFERATION OF NUCLEAR TECHNOLOGY

In recent months there has been an explosion of public interest in nuclear technology, partly sparked off by the publication of the Royal Commission Report on Nuclear Power and the Environment, and partly in response to Mr Benn's plea that there should be widespread debate on the subject. Awareness that a Government decision may be imminent on whether or not to start the next stage of the nuclear power programme by building fast breeder reactors has no doubt also been a factor in keeping the subject in the news. Whatever the reasons, hardly a day passes without some mention of the topic in the newspapers, and it may therefore be useful to have a broad, non-technical review of the issues from a Christian perspective.

The World Council of Churches has already produced two major studies on nuclear technology, one in preparation for, and the other resulting from, a Conference held in June 1975, at Sigtuna in Sweden. A number of individual churches have mounted their own studies. For instance, the Church of Scotland held a Conference in August 1976, under the title Infinite Potential or Infinite Risk?, which came to broadly the same conclusions as the United States National Council of Churches of Christ in proposing a moratorium on further developments until the issues and the alternatives to nuclear

This chapter was originally a presidential address to the British Group of the Council on Christian Approaches to Defence and Disarmament, Nov. 1976.

power are better understood. The W.C.C. was more cautious in its general conclusions: 'Our group cannot put forward categorical recommendations. It would not feel justified in either entirely rejecting, nor in whole-heartedly recommending large-scale use of nuclear energy.' One could scarcely be more judicious than that!

A factor inhibiting many from taking part in the debate may be fear about the technical complexity of the subject. The Royal Commission Report is admirably clear and introduces its main themes in a style which should be reasonably comprehensible to those without specialist scientific knowledge. But there is no denying the fact that technical considerations are of crucial importance in any informed ethical discussion. Ethics is not a study in vague generalities, but must take account of the actual complexity of things as they are.

This is not to say, however, that there can be no simplification. Indeed, my aim in this paper is to try to tease out the underlying issues of principle, and set them within as broad a context as possible. It is by scrutinizing the value judgements underlying complex choices, and by trying to assess these within the context of God's world and his purposes, that the Christian thinker can make his best contribution to the current debate.

During the summer of 1976 I visited the British Nuclear Fuels Re-processing Plant at Windscale, and ended the day by leading a discussion between some sixty or so church members employed in and around the Windscale Plant. The discussion achieved a minor breakthrough in that it was the first time that the exponents of very different views on nuclear energy had met there in reasoned argument; the success was largely due, it seems, to the fact that the context was deliberately made as broad as possible, and so lifted above the level of local politics. The immediate pressures were strong. It was obvious, for example, that there were many local fears of pollution on the one hand, or unemployment on the other. There was also a certain defensiveness among staff employed in the plant about the criticisms to which they were subjected in the press and by bodies like Friends of the Earth, and there was clearly no wish that Windscale should become another Aldermaston.

It became possible to face the issues constructively when we stopped arguing about minor degrees of pollution and infinitesimal risks, and tried to think instead what the world might be like in thirty or forty years' time when there could be as many as three thousand fast breeder reactors meeting a major proportion of the world's energy needs. It is at that stage in development that questions about the maintenance of standards in work which would by then have become routine, begin to become serious. Those with no doubts about our present nuclear installations may well be fearful of the time when the stimulus of a pioneering phase in development is over, and the motivation for safety-consciousness has declined. On the other hand, those employed in the industry were quick to point out how favourably their record compared with those of other dangerous industries, and they wondered why nuclear technology was especially singled out and subject to such unusually stringent standards. It was clear, however, that even a long-term look at the issues in terms of safety did not get to the root of the matter.

Our discussion led us to see that the underlying choices are social, ethical, and political. What kind of a society do we want to bequeath to future generations, bearing in mind that we now stand at a kind of watershed in technological development? Two rivers, originating at the same point and running down different sides of the mountain, may flow into quite different seas.

The Main Technical Considerations

Before looking at the broad social issues, though, I must first summarize the main technical considerations entailed in the choice which has to be made:

1. Future Energy Requirements

Everybody agrees that in twenty or thirty years' time the gap between energy consumption and the energy produced from conventional fossil fuels is going to be uncomfortably wide. There is no agreement, though, on how wide it is going to be, nor on the possible scale of future requirements. In its evidence to the Royal Commission the U.K. Atomic Energy Authority predicted a sevenfold increase in energy consumption between 1975 and 2030. It estimated that during that period the proportion of total electricity consumption generated by nuclear power would need to rise from 9.5% to 97%. The Royal Commission questioned these figures and proposed an alternative strategy in which consumption would only rise by 40% during the period, nuclear energy providing about 30% of the total. The Commission suggested that this modest increase could be achieved by a much more efficient use of energy and without drastic cutbacks in the rate of economic growth. It made a particular point of the inefficiency of electricity generation, an inefficiency inherent in the process, but which could be substantially reduced if the heat now dissipated by power stations was used, for example, for district heating schemes. This would entail siting power stations near centres of population.

The so-called Marshall Report on Energy Research and Development in the United Kingdom set out seven possible scenarios covering the next twenty-five years, and concluded that at an annual growth in energy consumption of 2.4% nuclear energy would be indispensable, but that at a 1.1% growth rate it would not be needed up till the year 2000, but thereafter would almost certainly be needed by 2025.

Differences of opinion of this order, of which these are only a few examples and in which so much depends upon one's initial assumptions, mean that no firm forecasts are possible. What is certain, however, is that on a world scale the consumption of energy is going to increase vastly. At present the energy consumption per capita in the United States is the equivalent of 11,500 kilogrammes of coal per annum. For Bangladesh the figure is 32; Western Europe has an average of around 4,000; otherwise, the only countries in the world which exceed 1,000 are Japan, Kuwait, and Israel. On any reasonable assumptions about world development, the energy needs of the majority of less favoured countries are going to increase many times. Since this development will be taking place during a period when the price of fossil fuels will be rising, there will be strong pressures in favour of using nuclear energy. Fast breeder reactors in particular will have enormous attractions, since their highly efficient use of uranium as their basic fuel could mean virtual self-sufficiency in energy terms for countries which process them and can do the necessary re-processing. This would in turn provide a certain security against inflation.

In the long-term, the dream of unlimited energy supplies depends on the successful exploitation of nuclear fusion. The hope is that the process might be free of long-term radio-active products, and use as its fuel an isotope of hydrogen which is present in enormous quantities in sea-water. And an extremely potent dream it is likely to be. The appropriate technology may not be ready for thirty years or more, if ever, but countries with limited energy supplies would need strong alternative reasons if they are not to pursue this as their ultimate goal.

2. Risks

It is convenient to think of these in three broad categories:
(a)   *The dangers inherent in routine operation.* There is no reason seriously to doubt the assurances given by those in the nuclear industry that at present the risk of any escape of radio-active materials from one of their plants is very small, as is the risk of a major catastrophe. Radio-activity has the advantage of being easy to monitor, and I believe that the industry is right to contrast its extremely high standards with those in other potentially dangerous fields.

However, as installations multiply, and as the potentially more dangerous fast breeder reactor comes into widespread use, the risks will multiply too. In these circumstances the degree of commitment and self-discipline required among those engaged in the industry will be enormous. It is a safe working rule to assume that any accident, however unlikely in theory, will eventually happen if there is any scope left for human error.

We rightly demand extremely high standards of safety in the nuclear industry because of the nature of the risk. The results of explosions, or of the release of pollutants, in other industries can be devastating in the short-term, but there is nothing comparable to the possible long-term effects of any major release of radio-activity. High standards are also demanded when the general public is at risk, in addition to those actually employed in the industry concerned. It also seems that risks are psychologically less acceptable when those exposed to them have no control over them; thus individuals will take risks with their own lives when driving a car, which would not be tolerated in a bus, and still less in a train where the driver is even more remote from the passengers. In the case of nuclear energy, a risk over which future generations might have no control for thousands of years seems particularly abhorrent.

On the other hand, human beings are risk-taking creatures, and although the risks in nuclear processes seem peculiarly sinister, they are, nevertheless, well understood – perhaps better understood than many which are accepted much more casually. Furthermore, if the nuclear programme were to be abandoned, and reliance placed on other sources of energy, there could well be risks entailed in its use, of which at present we have no conception. The suggestion in a recent book that the world might have a hydrogen economy by using sunlight to electrolyse water, filled a nuclear scientist with whom I was talking with horror. His reaction was that he would rather work on a nuclear pile any day than run his house or his car on bottled hydrogen. Moreover, even if a massive extraction of solar energy was possible, say by using the Sahara as a giant generating station, nobody knows what effects such installations might have on world climate. In other words, there are risks entailed whatever we do, and I do not myself believe that the risks inherent in the routine use of nuclear energy count decisively against it.

(b) *The dangers of pollution by radio-active waste.* The Royal Commission Report concluded that it would not be advisable to embark on a programme of nuclear expansion without further research into the means for disposing of long-term radio-active waste. Some waste products remain active for a very long time, running into thousands or even tens of thousands of years, and for a considerable part of that time they may generate sufficient heat to make special provision for cooling them essential. During my visit to Windscale I was allowed to clamber over one of the storage tanks in process of construction, where liquid waste will be stored until something better can be found to do with it. Each tank is a huge stainless steel structure with seven independent cooling systems which will have to be kept operational for an unforeseeable number of years. The row of tanks already filled and sealed up in their concrete containers was a vivid reminder that the problem of waste disposal does not only belong to the future.

It is true that various other means of disposal are being actively explored. The most promising of these involves solidifying the residues in glass, and burying them under the sea-bed in some part of the ocean where the geological formations are known to be stable. Even this method of disposal, however, can not provide a complete guarantee of protection against pollution over the long periods of time during which some of the waste will remain active.

It has been pointed out that the management of waste over periods of thousands of years demands a longevity in human institutions which none have so far attained. An American nuclear physicist has written: 'We have relatively little problem in dealing with wastes if we can assume that there will always be intelligent people around to cope with eventualities we have not thought of. . . .' In the same article he went on to point out that commitment to nuclear power is a commitment for ever, comparable in importance to primitive man's commitment to agriculture. Once the step was taken, and human institutions had been built, which depended on agriculture for their survival, there was no going back.

If this seems a large decision for a relatively unprepared world to take within the next few years, it is worth reiterating that whatever the decision, the problem is with us now and will remain with us for the foreseeable future. The waste from existing nuclear power plants, which is alarming enough in itself, is dwarfed by the large quantities of waste created as a result of nuclear weapons' programmes. It has been calculated that there is already ten times as much waste in existence as will be produced by any conceivable expansion of civil programmes during the next twenty years.

Apart from radio-active waste, there are other pollution problems connected with the generation of electricity in nuclear power stations, and the reliance on electricity as the major source of power. The most troublesome of these is likely to be heat pollution; approximately three times as much energy has to be dissipated as heat as is converted into electricity. The re-siting of power stations so that some of this available heat could be used directly in central heating systems, would run counter to the policy of siting nuclear power stations well away from centres of population. On the other hand, to site all the reactors on desolate coasts and to use the sea for cooling would create environmental disadvantages of another kind.

Pollution, in other words, is a major problem to which no definitive answers have yet been given. However, there is no reason to suppose that acceptable solutions will never be found, and the Royal Commission was surely right to conclude that there is a case for slowing down nuclear development until more research has been done on the subject of waste disposal, but that this is not a reason for abandoning the programme entirely.

(c) *Military risks.* These have received a lot of publicity recently, especially in relation to possible terrorist activities.

Risks from terrorism arise mainly because nuclear power plants are enormously expensive, would be difficult to protect in large numbers, and could be used as a powerful bargaining counter in a successful terrorist raid. The potential danger from damage or destruction, as well as the damage to the national economy, might make it very hard for any Government to hold out against terrorist demands.

In wartime the risks would be similar, with the added disadvantage of a highly-centralized energy supply which would presumably be a first target for enemy raids.

There has been much debate about the possible dangers resulting from movements of plutonium from re-processing plants to reactors, and it has been suggested that transport could be hijacked, or small quantities of plutonium spirited away for the manufacture of nuclear weapons. No doubt this is theoretically possible, but the difficulties would be formidable, and it has been argued that a determined group of terrorists would stand a much better chance of manufacturing or obtaining a successful bomb by stealing from military installations rather than civil ones.

Be that as it may, it is obvious that security must play a large part in any nuclear programme. A Friends of the Earth pamphlet has painted an alarming picture of the kind of police state which might develop as the result of the elaborate security precautions and screening procedures which any wide-scale commitment to nuclear power would necessitate. It seems to me, however, that the largest threat from nuclear installations resides in the fact that governments which are committed to nuclear technology can, if they wish, manufacture nuclear weapons. So long as the world is content to live with nuclear weaponry, the military risks created by nuclear power stations, though important, remain secondary. It is therefore difficult to counter the argument that those who have learnt to live with the bomb ought not to be too fastidious about the fast breeder reactor.

The risks I have so far described are real and serious, and there are those who feel that the world's need for additional sources of energy would have to be even more pressing than it now appears to be in order to justify running them. On the other hand, it can be claimed that all the risks are of a type which advancing societies have found themselves capable of handling, and that the alternatives are even more hazardous.

The disagreement points to the deeper questions of values underlying the mainly technical issues which have so far been considered. I return, therefore, to the basic question with which I started, namely, what kind of a society do we want?

One aspect of this larger question was pinpointed by the Chairman of the Royal Commission, Sir Brian Flowers, at the National Energy Conference held in June 1976. He said: 'We believe that nobody should rely for something as basic as energy on a process that produces in quantity a by-product as dangerous as plutonium.' The significance of that remark lies in the phrase 'as basic as energy'. The argument, in other words, is not about a fringe benefit, however desirable, but about the resource on which the whole of an industrial society depends, and which therefore deeply influences the character of that society. An Indian physicist has written:

Scratch any piece of technology and you will find the values and aims of a society it was designed to serve. For technology is like genetic material – it carries with it the code of the society which conceived it. This is why the choice of technology is such a crucial decision in the developing countries today. The kind of society and the kind of environment which they will create depends to a large extent on what technology they choose for the job of development.

Nuclear energy not only creates new forms of society by enabling industrial and economic expansion to be continued into the foreseeable future. It also implies a certain kind of society, in that it requires a broad technical base to support the highly advanced technology on which that society's primary resource must depend.

This consideration about the kind of society implied by nuclear technology may be equally valid if and when fusion reactors become a practical possibility. It is often assumed that the problematic nature of nuclear technology arises mainly from the risks associated with a fast breeder programme, and that these will virtually disappear when fusion power comes on the scene. The social implications, however, will remain. These will differ in character, though, depending on whether workable fusion reactors turn out to be very large, or whether fusion by means of laser beams leads to the development of small localized power plants.

Some Social Implications Of A Nuclear Energy Programme

1. In developed countries
An expanding nuclear programme might provide a strong temptation to suppose that the general rate of economic expansion in developed countries could continue without interruption. Whether or not this would be tolerable in terms of other resources besides energy, and whether continued expansion would simply increase the disparities between rich and poor countries is one of the major social and political questions facing the industrialized world today. The World Council of Churches' studies on this theme have developed the idea of 'the sustainable society' within which the rate of expansion has been reduced either to zero, or to a figure which could be sustained for the foreseeable future.

It is possible to envisage a sustainable society which makes use of nuclear energy, and to that extent decisions about the one are separable from decisions about the other. Nevertheless, the fact that far-reaching decisions have to be made about nuclear energy provides a unique opportunity to think deeply about long-term aims for society, at a time when the risks of continued expansion are clearly seen, and the doubts about energy supplies have not yet been silenced by a massive commitment of capital to a particular solution. No solution is without its hazards, and the move towards a sustainable society, with or without nuclear energy, would carry particularly severe social ones. Would people stand for a slowing down of our present social economic machine? What would be the effect of a gradually decreasing growth rate in terms of jobs, standards of living and the general health and security of society? Are longings for a simpler life-style confined to those who have already had their fair share of this world's goods, and would a cutback now seem like the ultimate betrayal to those who have just begun to get their feet on the ladder of prosperity? Are we caught in a technological trap from which there is no escape except into more technology? If it is claimed that it is possible to say 'no' to continued expansion, and to the nuclear programme which would have to undergird it, we have to face the fact that, in the words of John Francis, 'there is not a single example in which mankind has currently succeeded in holding a rapidly advancing technology at arm's length', mainly because the political and economic incentives for continuing in our present direction are too strong.

2. In developing countries
The same long-term considerations apply in developing countries as in developed ones. There is the added complication, however, that some developing countries see nuclear power as a guarantee of their own independence. For example, a spokesman from Latin America, writing about the exploitation of coal and oil by the industrialized nations adds: 'That history is not going to be repeated in respect of nuclear energy. This means that we are not prepared any more to just wait and see what the powerful nations are going to do. . . .

Nuclear energy has really inspired the idea of self-reliance in the technological sector that is now spreading all over the world.'[1] He goes on to say that developing nations are quite prepared to make their own mistakes.

Such independence, of course, if achieved would be relative, not least in a cultural sense. I have already made the point that to import an advanced technology inevitably means importing the cultural background which sustains it. India's programme, which was begun only a year after independence, was pursued at a time of great social need, both as a visible symbol of independence and also as a means of stimulating indigenous science. India also illustrates how a nuclear power programme cannot be separated from a weapons' programme. It seems clear that any attempt to force such a separation on developing nations would be deeply resented. It would strike at the heart of the very self-reliance, both economic and political, which the nuclear programme would be designed to achieve.

One of the alarming features of the nuclear age would lie in the concentration of political power it would encourage, and this fact must be set against all talk of independence. Does independence mean independence for people, or for their political rulers? We have already seen in Britain how the centralization of energy supplies puts enormous power in the. hands of a very small number of people, whether the legitimate government, or those determined to influence it. There is also the point already mentioned about the degree of surveillance needed over nuclear installations and the transport of nuclear fuel, and the political implications which flow from this. The international dimension of nuclear control might, if handled wisely, lead to a greater sense of world community and a more just distribution of resources. Unfortunately, it could just as easily lead to an increasing gulf between rich and poor, and a heightened authoritarianism.

1. In a submission to a W. C. C. Hearing on Nuclear Energy.

Conclusion

In the end the choices made by individuals and by nations are much influenced by ill-formulated beliefs about human nature, and it is on this level that Christian insights can perhaps be of most help in clarifying the issues. Are human beings resilient enough to cope with the unprecedented problems of a nuclear age and the permanent commitment which this would entail? Alternatively, is this possibly our last opportunity to reverse the current trends? Which is more fundamental as a type of Christian response – thrusting creativeness or a humble acknowledgment of human limitations?

The concept of stewardship has been fruitful in recent Christian discussions on these themes. It implies a sense of responsibility concerning the resources entrusted to us, as in the parable of the servants who doubled their capital, while denying that human ambitions can be the sole criterion for deciding how they should be used.

My own belief is that we have for too long identified the creativeness for which man was made, with scientific and technological advance, and now need to place greater emphasis on the kind of moral and spiritual restraints within which it must be exercised. At the heart of Christian affirmation of the world there is an element of holding back, supremely exemplified in the central Christian doctrine of Incarnation. Within the overflowing of divine love there was a scaling-down to human limitations – 'Being in the form of God . . . he humbled himself, taking the form of a servant.' Love shows itself as much in what it does not do as in what it does.

Is there a clue here about the basic frame of mind in which to approach these enormously complex decisions? The expression of doubts about the nuclear power programme may be an important reminder of the need to recover a sense of restraint in many other features of our social and political life. It is thus not inconceivable that there could be a moral feedback in what would be an undeniably courageous political decision.

This is not to deny, however, that a decision by the United Kingdom not to proceed with an expanded nuclear programme, could be made on purely pragmatic political grounds. I believe it could be a sensible decision even if, as seems likely, many other countries choose differently. In the first place, by forgoing a fast breeder programme the United Kingdom could be free to put capital into the development of other energy resources which might, at a later stage, be of great benefit not only to ourselves but to developing countries in other parts of the world, or even to other industrialized nations if unsuspected snags appear on the nuclear front. Britain is uniquely well-equipped to pursue such alternatives in view of our large reserves of conventional fuels. Secondly, if in the end attempts to develop these alternatives fail, it would almost certainly be possible to buy the appropriate nuclear technology at a later stage, in view of the strong likelihood that some countries at least will pursue fast breeder programmes. Thirdly, the policy of buying at a later stage might make commercial sense in the light of the organizational difficulties in the present British nuclear industry. Lord Hinton, former head of the Central Electricity Generating Board, writing in a recent edition of *New Scientist*, has said as much, though no doubt more as a bargaining counter than as a serious statement of policy. The implication is, though, that even a man as closely identified with reactor development as he was, is prepared to entertain the idea that Britain might opt out at this stage.

My own conclusion is that we should do so. It is not often that a decision of this magnitude, which is above party politics and which will deeply affect the future of the nation, can unite those who are worried on a purely technological level with those who see deeper social, ethical and ultimately religious issues at stake.

Postscript

This essay was written before the Windscale Enquiry, which succeeded in allaying some fears about nuclear energy, though by no means all of them. If I had been writing it now I would also have drawn attention to recent anxieties about carbon dioxide build-up in the atmosphere, as a result of continuing reliance on the consumption of fossil fuels. Whether such a build-up could lead to long-term, and potentially disastrous, climatic changes is still very fiercely debated. But there is certainly a new question mark over the policy of just going on as we are.

These considerations are not, in my view, sufficient to tip the balance in favour of the fast breeder reactor. There is, however, a strong case for continuing to develop the present generation of fission reactors, if only to ensure that enough expert staff are kept in employment.

8
THE ETHICAL DIMENSION IN ENERGY POLICY

It is difficult enough for individuals, and even more difficult for governments and nations, to tackle ethical issues head-on. Ethical assumptions are generally implicit in practical decisions, but more often than not do their work without conscious recognition. To analyse these assumptions, therefore, and ask questions about the relationship between different value judgements may not make the actual business of decision-making any easier. Thus there is no chance of complex questions about energy policy being answered by a simple direct appeal to ethical principles. This does not mean, however, that the ethical dimension can and should be ignored. Fundamental questions about values are not made any less important by the fact that they are difficult to answer. The values expressed in particular decisions are likely to have a longer-lasting influence than the obvious consequences of the decisions themselves. The attempt to expose them provides a perspective from which practical policies can be criticized, and introduces new possibilities of changing both the values and the decisions.

A. N. Whitehead, in his classic *Adventures of Ideas* made the point that potentially explosive ideas may lie dormant for many centuries:

They start as speculative suggestions in the minds of a small, gifted group. They acquire a limited application to

This chapter was originally a Paper prepared for a Council for Science and Society working party on Energy policy, May 1978.

life at the hands of various sets of leaders with special
functions in the social structure. A whole literature arises
which explains how inspiring is the general idea, and how
slight need be its effect in disturbing a comfortable society.
Some transition has been produced by the agency of the
new idea. But on the whole, the social system has been
inoculated against the full infection of the new principle.
It takes its place among the interesting notions which have
a limited application.

He went on to describe how the generation which actually
puts the ideas into effect is not necessarily wiser or superior
to its predecessors. What happens is simply that conditions
change 'so that what is possible now may not have been
possible then'.

Whitehead was writing about the abolition of slavery, but
his remarks are relevant to the general, and still only partially
formed, ideas about environmentalism and social change,
which act as one pole of the energy debate. Environmentalism
has had striking local successes. Its growth as an idea has
been extremely rapid, but its theoretical basis is still weak,
and the process of changing popular attitudes and assumptions has scarcely begun. A good illustration of its embyronic
state is the current confusion about the aims of the various
opponents of nuclear energy. Some see the anti-nuclear lobby
as a lever for bringing about much more fundamental changes
in society, a decentralized 'soft energy' future as opposed to
our present commitment to high technology and centralized,
capital-intensive industries. Others are concerned more with
the balance of risks inherent in different energy policies, and
emphasize the environmental, as well as the military, hazards
of an expanded nuclear programme. Others, it appears, simply climb onto a convenient anti-establishment bandwaggon
for what are basically political motives.

Such confusions can be treated cynically, and the enthusi-
asms of environmentalists can be dismissed as a luxury,
enjoyed by those who live in prosperous countries, which

would not survive real shortages. On the other hand, they can be seen as the preliminary gropings of a powerful idea in the making, which has still not reached the point of political take-off, but which is becoming increasingly available for use when conditions are right. Long-term decisions about energy policy need to take into account the fact that human ideas, no less than technical developments, have a long lead-time, which is why it is important to set present confusions on the subject of environmentalism within an historical context. Are we witnessing a slow change in attitudes concerning man's responsibility for his environment which, at the appropriate moment, will be seen to justify radical social transformations, and make them appear less painful than they do now? Or will the idealism which tries to express itself through environmentalist movements, be permanently frustrated by rising social and economic expectations? or give place to a different kind of idealism? And if it is frustrated in competitive Western societies, does it follow that developing countries, with their different cultural traditions, would necessarily face the same conflicts?

If rising expectations seem at present likely to prevail in Western policies, the question then has to be asked, how long this process can continue, bearing in mind the changes which will be needed in the world economic order if there is to be a stable future, recognized as just; bearing in mind also the finiteness of the world's other basic resources besides energy. At some point, sooner or later, the curve of rising expectations must flatten, and less extravagant ideas about human fulfilment must take priority. The question is, When? And what kind of preparation for this transition is it appropriate to make now? In part the answers must depend on personal judgements about the strength, validity, and likely growth rate of environmentalist ideas; in part they entail political judgements about the kind of social and international pressures and crises which might force rapid change.

From these general considerations about the future character of society, it may be helpful to isolate three more specific questions in which the ethical dimension is of particular significance:

1. The question of time-scale

It is widely assumed that each generation has obligations towards posterity, but there is no agreement on the time-scale of these obligations, or the extent to which it is reasonable to jeopardize the future for the sake of the present, or vice versa.

In a stable, relatively static, society it is easy to see how justice is served if each generation leaves its successors with as many, or more, freedoms and opportunities as it has itself enjoyed. The time-scale need not extend beyond one's own children and grandchildren, and the sense of obligation arises out of a concern for those with whom there are direct and personal links.

In a society marked by rapid growth, both in terms of population and in the consumption of finite resources, the equation is different, and it is made more complex by the fact that major decisions may have to be made a generation before they can be implemented. The full consequences of some of these decisions, e.g. the disposal of radio-active waste, may have to be considered on a time-scale longer than that of recorded history. In such a society the bequest which each generation makes to its successors has to be evaluated as a balanced whole. Thus it is possible to argue that the long-term problems of radio-active waste are part of a package which includes a long-term commitment to a high-technology future, which is likely to have avoided the traumas of social change through energy shortage, but which is exposed to high risks of nuclear warfare. The benefits of preserving the present structures and aspirations of civilized life might be thought to justify the risks, in that they include the provision of the wherewithal to cope with them.

Others might argue that social stability can be bought at too high a price if it entails the squandering of non-renewable resources, or the commitment of future generations to reliance on very advanced technology for meeting their basic needs. But it has to be asked of those who advocate heroic restraint, whether there are not proven dangers in trying to sacrifice the present for the sake of the future.

Compromise packages which provide for reasonable restraint and maximum flexibility would seem the best way forward, but it is likely that these will succeed only if the time-scale is kept relatively short. Restraint exercised to protect those a thousand years hence, who might possibly suffer from radio-active contamination, would soon begin to seem unreal when energy shortages began to bite. On the other hand, restraint which has obvious benefits for one's children and grandchildren has a stronger motivation to sustain it. Longer-term considerations demand reasonable precautions, but not unreasonable sacrifices.

2. The question of risks

Life is inherently fragile; people are inherently fallible; all energy-producing processes contain dangers, greater or less. It is therefore impossible to have an energy policy which is devoid of risks, though these may be distributed in different ways as between the primary producers, the processors, the consumers, and those without any direct involvement.

An analysis of risks from an ethical standpoint would need to concern itself with the type or scale of risk in relation to the benefits conferred, and more particularly with the question, Who suffers what risk for whose benefit?

The risks of a large-scale commitment to nuclear energy, for instance, range from the, admittedly minute, risk of direct radio-active contamination to the long-term risk of storage, from the risks of mining uranium to the risk of a major disaster, from the risks of lowered safety standards through the widespread proliferation of nuclear plants to the risk of nuclear war through the increased availability of plutonium. Some of these risks affect only the people who have agreed to run them as a result of their choice of work. Others affect everybody.

In weighing them against each other, and against the enormous benefits of nuclear energy, some sort of scale of importance has to be devised. It has already been suggested that, in relation to the long-term shortage of waste, reasonable precautions rather than infallible guarantees of safety are the best one can hope for. This is because remote risks to remote generations are unlikely to seem as important as the direct dangers, however small, to people who live in the vicinity of a nuclear power station. Directness and immediacy count more in popular opinion than subtle statistical considerations, and it is hard to weigh up the risks and benefits of a legacy to future generations.

But in an ethical calculus it would seem that the major risks in any enterprise should be borne by those who have chosen to take them, and by those most likely to benefit from them. This would be a factor to put in the balance against bequeathing hidden, and possibly unknown, dangers to our descendants. It is also relevant when comparing, say, the deaths caused by coal-mining with the deaths from accidental radio-active leakage.

The balance of risks should also include social factors. Dangers to life and limb have to be set against the long-term unhappiness and possibilities of social unrest which might be entailed by a serious energy shortage. There are also questions about the structuring of society, security measures, and curtailment of freedom implied by different policies. In most hierarchies of value, life and health count for more than less tangible social values. But this is not an absolute priority, or else there would be no wars. Considerations of scale also enter into the calculus.

3. *The question of justice*
Energy is a world problem. In a just world where unified

policies were practicable, a wide variety of energy resources could be co-ordinated in ways appropriate to local needs. In the world as it is, there is an imbalance of resources which could become dangerously destabilizing, and which there is not yet the political will to correct.

A general ethical concern to create a just and sustainable society might be given political assistance by a sufficiently skilful handling of the nuclear energy issue. It is widely accepted that security, both in the actual production of nuclear energy and in its possible abuse through the proliferation of nuclear weapons, presupposes strong and effective means of international control. The growth of an international and dedicated corps of scientists and technicians who might in the future have a major part in controlling and maintaining one of the world's main supplies of energy, could do much to ensure fairer distribution and better co-operation between nations. On the other hand, if it is mishandled, nuclear energy might further divide the world into destructively competitive groups with vested interests in expansion for the wrong motives, and could increase the gap between the 'haves' and the 'have nots'.

A second factor which could be made to work in the interests of justice between the nations, is the realization that the balance of the world's energy resources is likely to shift decisively when the oil runs out. Put simply, if the world of the future is going to have to depend more on sunlight, then Africa has more of it than Europe.

Justice within nations is also influenced by energy policies. To take an obvious example, the effect of a nuclear programme on a semi-industrialized country is almost inevitably to put power in the hands of a minority and to heighten social inequalities. The appropriate technology movement is as much concerned with constructive social development as with the best use of resources, but even it has been criticized for sometimes creating more social problems than it solves. In developed industrial countries, too, pricing policies for different kinds of energy, or programmes of energy conservation, can easily bear most hardly on those least equipped to respond to them flexibly.

Within nations, politicians are usually sensitive to this kind of issue. But between nations the pursuit of justice has a long way to go. Politicians who can harness it to the world's need for energy will be building the best foundation for the future.

9

TECHNOLOGY AND POLITICS: ETHICAL REFLECTIONS ON THE ARMS RACE

Do technical developments determine policies or do policies indicate the needed technical developments? Or is the relationship between the two much more complex than such a simple opposition might suggest? Some complain of the extent to which policy-makers fail to make the best use of technical developments already available. Others point to the degree of ignorance, even in Government circles, of the development of new weapons until the results are presented as a *fait accompli*. Some see technology as a sinister force, increasingly independent of the political process, in that few except a small élite understand what they are doing. Others regard it as a normal part of being human; man is, and always has been, a toolmaker and the sophistication of his tools extends rather than diminishes him.

In such a highly charged debate I can do no more than try to clarify some of the issues, and point to some Christian insights which may be relevant in the limited context of weapons technology. But first a case has to be made that such insights can, and should, make a difference.

This chapter was originally a Paper prepared for the 1977 International Conference of the Council on Christian Approaches to Defence and Disarmament. First published in *Crucible*, Jan. 1978, as 'Technology and Politics'.

'Can implies ought'?

Technology is now such a dominant feature of the way of life in developed countries, and the rate of technological advance is so rapid, that it is easy to succumb to a belief in its inevitability. The mere possibility of some technical innovation invites the presupposition that in due course it will be tried out in practice. Once something becomes thinkable, people will go on thinking it, and even if the originator of an idea takes it no further, the chances are that sooner or later someone else will. It has frequently been remarked that in the history of science ideas have their appropriate time, and many people may be on the verge of making the same discovery when a particular breakthrough comes.

There is no way, therefore, of putting a brake on creative thought or human invention, and in a competitive society the practical disadvantages of even trying to do so are obvious. Nor does the long history of opposition to scientific and technical advance offer much encouragement to those who feel that it ought to be possible to stop it. Yesterday's dangerous innovation becomes today's commonplace. A recent writer, commenting on the nuclear proliferation debate, has said: 'There is no single instance in which mankind has currently succeeded in holding a rapidly advancing technology at arm's length. . . .' Those who fear that our present technological momentum is a major, perhaps the major, factor in shaping the modern world, have solid reasons for doing so.

Control by debate

On the other hand, it constantly needs to be asserted that technology is a human enterprise, the result of human choices, and its advance is only inevitable if those who make the choices believe that they have no alternative. Over-emphasis on technological dominance creates self-fulfilling prophecies.

In fact there are many ways in which control can be, and is exercised, of which the most obvious is selective funding. The more sophisticated technology becomes, the greater its dependence on Government finance, and the greater the likelihood that political considerations will determine the choices. Too much political control may be as undesirable as too little and, since the reasons behind the decision-making at this level are often obscure, there is much to be said for devising some machinery for widespread public debate about controversial projects.

A report published by the Council for Science and Society on *Superstar Technologies* is sub-titled 'The problem of monitoring technologies in those instances where technical competence is monopolised by a small number of institutions committed to the same interest'. Its particular concern is with safety and scientific standards in highly sophisticated technological enterprises where informed external criticism is hard to obtain. What it says about the importance of public debate at an early conceptual stage in such projects surely applies with even greater force in the closed world of defence technology. But timing is of the essence in effective criticism. If criticism comes too late, the investment already made in an idea is likely to silence it.

A good example of the way in which public opinion can nevertheless have a decisive effect, even at a late stage in matters of military technology, was the disquiet in America over ecological warfare in Vietnam. In throwing doubts on the legitimacy of the war, it probably contributed substantially to its outcome. Whether such weapons will ever be used again remains to be seen, but the fact that certain applications of science to warfare create acute controversy, while others have alreay been banned, is a striking proof that the political control of technology can be effective. However, controversies tend to be confined to new technologies. Beyond the conceptual stage there may be a further crucial period during the introduction of, say, a new weapons system, when public opinion is of the utmost importance. Thereafter, what has become familiar is likely to go on being accepted.

Weapons presuppose a context for their own use. A new weapon is not merely a technological device, but has built into it a series of military, political and ethical assumptions which do not follow automatically from the technological advances which have made it possible. The neutron warhead, in which a substantial proportion of the blast from a nuclear explosion is transformed into short-lived lethal radiation, presupposes a military context in which it is more desirable to kill people than to knock down buildings. It could be used, for instance, to stop a massive tank advance, and its attractiveness to defence experts lies in its supposed effectiveness, and relative cleanness, as a tactical weapon. We are told that the necessary technology has been available for twenty years or more. The decision to build it is a political one. The ethical controversy it has aroused has focused, unwisely in my view, on the inhumanity of devising a weapon which is especially efficient in destroying human flesh. More effective arguments against it, as I shall indicate later, rest on the psychology of deterrence.

War, and the threat of war, stimulate technology, and it is almost certain that without this stimulus the two largest technological enterprises of recent years, the space programme and the development of nuclear energy, would not have taken place. Technology, on the other hand, changes the character of war by making it more devastating and more impersonal. It thus creates a paradox in which the moral responsibility for the effects of war is increased, while the sense of personal responsibility in actual fighting is diminished. Serious talk of casualties in terms of millions is only possible for those who are distant enough from the consequencies of their actions.

The appeal to ethical insight

Within this complex interaction between the pressures of technological invention and political realism the voice of those who appeal to ethical insights may seem very feeble. Yet it is a basic fact of human nature that men even, or perhaps especially, when they are making hard decisions about intractable problems, seek to justify themselves by reference to principles and values on which these decisions are based. The principles may be wrong-headed or misapplied, and frequently become distorted in the actual course of a conflict, but the fact remains that some kind of moral legitimacy is sought even for the most horrific actions. The critical assessment of principles and values, therefore, is far from being a marginal activity. Most human action has an ethical dimension, and it is interesting to observe the extent to which this is now recognized in areas which, until quite recently, would have been regarded as value-free. A general growth of uncertainty about the desirability of unlimited scientific and technological advance is one symptom of this new ethical awareness. And the most striking contemporary example of it is the current debate on the proliferation of nuclear energy in which scientific, technical, political, international, social and ethical considerations are inextricably interwoven. Christians have no ready-made set of principles from which answers to such problems can be deduced. Recent discussions, held under the auspices of the World Council of Churches on the subject of Science and Technology for Human Development, have stressed the ambiguity of technical advance, its potential for both good and evil, and have also illustrated the delicate balance between short-term practical decision-making, and long-term hopes and ideals. In fact Christian ethics has always moved between the two poles of what is practicable at a given time and radical criticism of basic principles. No Christian can ignore the Sermon on the Mount. Equally, no Christian, especially if he carries social responsibilities, can live as if his more mundane obligations were of no account. The contribution of Christian insights to ethical discussion is thus made on various levels. On some levels the territory has been well mapped and old practical guidelines, such as the

Just War doctrine, still retain some usefulness. On other levels Christian insights may set the tone of a discussion without suggesting any specific action. A stress on human sinfulness, for instance, may serve as a corrective to naive optimism; alternatively the message of Christian hope may provide encouragement to grasp opportunities for constructive change, and prevent political realism from lapsing into fatalism.

Three Christian contributions

Specific Christian insights in a particular field like weapons technology are harder to be certain about, but I tentatively suggest three:

1. The first is a general criticism of the belief that human problems can be solved by technological means – the so-called 'technical fix'. Another report published by the Council for Science and Society on *Harmless Weapons* (i.e. the use of sophisticated devices in the control of civil disorder) makes the important point that the more such devices are used by the police, the more their relationship with the civil population is damaged, and the harder it becomes for their ultimate aim in preserving the peace to be achieved. The same may be true in war. In losing sight of the ultimate aim of military operations in trying to create a peaceful, just and sustainable world society, those who are placing their reliance on technological superiority may unwittingly betray the end by concentrating on the means.

War is fundamentally a human problem, not a technological one, and a major part of Christian witness in the face of war must be to concentrate attention on the human factors which cause it. And this implies abandoning the belief that the technological race between nations could or should ever be won.

2. Christian ethics has always made use of the notion of limits. In different ages and different circumstances the limits have been specified in different ways, but there is a persistent tradition that there are boundaries in human behaviour, which ought not to be crossed, whatever the provocation. The Just War tradition, with its principles of 'proportion' and 'discrimination' was an attempt to set limits on the use of military power. Though its main justification was theological, it can also be defended on non-religious commonsense grounds, which is perhaps why it has still managed to retain some influence.

Precise limits are difficult to define. Even so, the notion that limits exist can help to counteract the general tendency to drift in human affairs, which obscures the crossing of important boundaries. Those who see the limits more clearly than others can help to sharpen the consciences of those who feel themselves driven by practical necessity.

For instance, it is a serious question whether anything, however threatening, could justify a major nuclear war. Politically and ethically there is still a sharp dividing-line between nuclear and non-nuclear hostilities, and the risks of a nuclear holocaust are diminished so long as this dividing-line is maintained, and the psychological barrier against crossing it is high. In military terms, however, the psychological barrier has already been crossed by tactical nuclear weaponry, and there are military pressures to lower it still further. The neutron warhead is simply the latest step in a long progression, and will be justified on the grounds that its effectiveness as a potential killer makes the nuclear deterrent more credible. On the other hand it can equally well be argued that its very effectiveness, in damaging the psychological barrier, might increase the chances of a slide into all-out nuclear war. My own view is that this is one of the areas in which the Christian conscience ought to say 'No'; not by advocating any unrealistic abandonment of nuclear capability, but by stressing the unpredictable and irreversible consequences of crossing this particular ethical and psychological barrier, and by opposing policies which might have the effect of lowering it.

A related issue is the current debate about the proliferation of nuclear technology for peaceful purposes. There seems little chance of avoiding the spread of nuclear energy to many countries which have not hitherto had it, and there are strong grounds for claiming that it would not in any case be just to limit the rights of developing countries to its benefits. On the other hand, current debate about the development of breeder reactors which, if they were to become a main source of nuclear power, would inevitably lead to a large increase in the availability of weapons' grade plutonium, poses the question whether there is not here also a limit which ought not to be passed. Subsidiary arguments about the risks of nuclear technology, the disposal of radioactive waste and the safeguarding of nuclear installations, have created a climate of popular concern which, at least in Britain, would make a decision against the further development of breeder reactors politically possible. Such a decision might strengthen the ethical and psychological barriers against the otherwise seemingly inevitable spread of nuclear weaponry.

3. Christians must refuse to think about war in impersonal terms, just as they must oppose anything that belittles or destroys human relationships. Part of the crisis of Christian conscience over modern warfare lies not only in the devastation it can cause physically, but in the absence of the kind of personal relationships between combatants, which in other circumstances can impose their own restraints. Human value is destroyed, as well as individual human beings, and the consequent wounds go deeper.

It would be foolishly unrealistic to hope that greater technological sophistication could reverse the trend towards killing by remote control. However, there are compensating factors which might be recognized and exploited more fully, the most obvious of which is the growth of mass communications. Though combatants in modern war may never see each other, television can show it happening, and can illustrate its effects in highly personal terms. The influence of television on the outcome of the Vietnam war is a matter for debate, but it undoubtedly enabled very large numbers of people to identify themselves with the war to an extent which would not otherwise have been possible. And this in some measure, I believe, limited its destructiveness of human values.

Large abstract claims about the depersonalizing effects of modern technology achieve little. But sensitivity to the ways in which personal values are in fact over-ridden, and skilful use of the means provided by technology to enhance personal awareness, would seem to me a valid Christian response.

10

SCIENCE: A SIGN OF THE TIMES

I saw a chip the other day – not the kind that goes with fish. This was a silicon chip, one of the miniature computer circuits which, so the Prime Minister has told us, are now to be the subject of massive new investment. The chip itself was quite hard to see; it was tiny, like a grain of mustard seed. And like a grain of mustard seed, its possibilities for growth are staggering. It is a seed which could revolutionize our world.

This Advent we are trying to discern the signs of the times; and the question I have been asked is, what are the signs of God's activity in the world of science? In fact I am going to look at a few things happening in the borderland between science and technology, because it is these practical things which affect us first. I begin with silicon chips because their impact is going to be felt in a big way, very soon indeed.

More, and cheaper, and more complex computers are only just over the horizon. Did you know that a piece of computing which in 1960 might have cost £1,000, might now cost a penny? How many, I wonder, already possess their own calculators? Elaborate industrial processes which used to be done by complex machinery and skilled human operators, can now be done simply and reliably by electronics. There is no need for me to dwell on the consequences of widespread automation; enough people are worried about it already. But if you want an illustration of what this next phase in the industrial revolution can do, look at the thousands of digital

This chapter was originally a sermon preached at morning service on B.B.C. Radio 4 as part of an Advent course on 'The Signs of the Times', Dec. 1978. The Lesson was Mark 4.26–32.

watches in our shops. The other side of the picture, the side
which is not so obvious to us in this country, is the virtual
wiping out of the Swiss watch industry.

Massive industrial and social changes are coming – and
coming fast. To some they seem exciting, to others threatening. To some they carry the promise of eventual release from
boring, backbreaking, mind-stultifying work. To others they
open up awful prospects of perpetual unemployment, of lives
empty of significance because there is nothing useful for
people to do. Nothing useful? We could, of course, do a great
deal more for each other, caring for one another in ways
which no silicon chip could possibly compete with. But to see
things like that is going to entail a moral and spiritual revolution, as well as a technological one.

So what is God saying to us through this sign of the times?
As always, he gives us a challenge and a promise. The challenge is to find a meaning in human life, which does not
depend upon people being busy and slaving away at mindless
jobs. The challenge is to find ways of so organizing our world
that everyone can feel wanted even if work is reduced to a
minimum. The promise is that the challenge can be met,
because your worth and my worth does not depend upon our
commercial value; it does not depend upon what ordinarily
counts as success. Our worth lies deeper than that. It depends
on God's own love for us. It depends on the fact that he has
made us his children. And to know that is to have an inner
dignity which nothing can shake.

Put it another way. The silicon chip revolution, a revolution
in which much that human beings have formerly done and
thought can now be done for them, drives us to ask about the
things in life which are distinctively and irreducibly human.
God's question hammers at us – what are you? When you
have all the leisure you need, when you have been to Torre-
molinos and Disneyland, when you have watched the ump-
teenth showing of your favourite Hollywood classic on T.V.,
what are you living for? What are your spiritual roots? It is
a strange paradox that technological advance should drive us

back to basic spirituality.

As I read the signs of the times, God is pointing us to a vision of human life stripped of many of its burdens, free to concentrate on human love and care and relationship, free to explore the inner things of the spirit, free to develop capacities which only flower when time is not pressing us. Science, technology, can make us more human. The hope is always that they will. The driving force of science is the vision of a better, nobler life. But the signs need not point that way. Leisure could destroy us, as it tended to destroy those in the past who had too much of it. Computers are servants of humanity. They can extend human powers in ways which it is hard for most of us even to imagine, let alone come to terms with. In doing so they place upon us an immense burden of responsibility. Are we ready to bear it? To tackle not just the economic problems, but the human ones?

A second sign, a very different one, a baby born in Calcutta. There was only an insignificant paragraph in the newspapers, but I asked myself when I read it, why, in India of all places, doctors felt it right to produce the world's second test-tube baby.

I know the arguments in favour. Even in a country desperately struggling with the problems of over-population, the misery of a childless couple is not to be ignored. Even in a country hard put to it to provide the simplest medical care for millions of its people, medical research at the frontiers of knowledge and at the limits of technical expertise, must still go on. There is a momentum in scientific research which has to be sustained, and those who are caught up in it and are creating our future must not feel restricted by mundane thoughts of usefulness or appropriateness.

But there is such a thing as a sense of proportion. There are priorities. And to me that baby is a tragic symbol of priorities which have somehow gone terribly wrong. No doubt in this country there is more justification for such experiments; they are spurred on partly by the hope that one day tragic deformities in newborn babies will be a thing of the past. But even here there are doubts about priorities; there are long-term fears too about the more sinister possibilities of genetic tinkering. But let that be.

At the moment I see this test-tube baby as a sign of the way the scientific bandwaggon rolls relentlessly on; things are done, clever things, often spectacular things, simply because it is possible to do them. There are lots of examples. I know it is superficial and unfair to compare the costs of a space research programme with the resources needed to relieve desperate human poverty. Again, I understand how scientists in defence departments get caught up in the race to develop new forms of frightful weapons, while those who seek to build peace between nations constantly find their work overtaken by ingenious new threats. In fact, it is difficult to see how the growth of human knowledge and its applications can avoid swamping us with too much power, too fast and with too little sense of its moral implications. But I believe God is telling us to look at our priorities.

'The kingdom of God is like a man who scatters seed on the land . . .'; it 'sprouts and grows, how he does not know. The ground produces a crop by itself. . . .' Things go on mysteriously, even apart from human intervention. Science seems to have a life of its own. Knowledge and power grow and multiply. Obviously in actual practice it is human knowledge won by human skills, but it sometimes seems as if human beings were carried along irresistibly as new realms of discovery and exploitation are opened up. Until the harvest. Then comes judgement. What our cleverness has grown is judged by its fruits.

The mushroom cloud over Hiroshima was a sign of judgement. The scientists who had produced it went through agonies as they tried to come to terms with a new sense of responsibility for the powers they handled. I hope a new-born baby in Calcutta never comes to know itself as a sign of judgement. To its parents surely it is a sign of fulfilment and hope. At the right time and in the right place the work of scientists can bring enormous blessing. But sometimes, and for me this is one of the times, such achievements have a question mark over them, God asking us what kind of harvest we are working for, and where our priorities lie.

My third and last sign, and a much more familiar one, is the humble battery hen. The battery hen is what happens when scientifically-minded people begin to apply their minds to the problem of producing the maximum number of eggs and the maximum amount of chicken with the minimum waste and the least possible human labour. The result is cheap eggs, cheap chickens, and more people able to afford more food than they ever enjoyed before. Excellent – except for the hens. And this is where some doubts begin to creep in. What are we doing to creatures if we treat them simply and solely as egg-producing machines? Might there be something wrong with a style of animal husbandry, or with an attitude to nature as a whole, which treats them simply as things to be exploited?

It is not only hens. Nobody has invented a cow yet which works only a five-day week and allows its cowman to do the same, and so it is still possible for the cowman and his cows to enter into some sort of relationship, an echo of the old sense of partnership with nature, of working alongside God's creatures. But what about veal? No partnership there, just fattening flesh, broiler hens on four legs.

I do not mean to be sentimental; I am fully aware of the constraints on food producers – notice how the word seems more appropriate than 'farmers' – in a highly competitive world. But as we search for the signs of the times, it seems to me that this changed relationship towards the world of nature, changed in the very activity, animal care, which once brought man and nature closest together, is a sign of much else that science has done for us and to us. For us – its benefits are all around us and on our tables. To us – has there been a certain deadening of heart, a cutting loose from old ties and obligations?

Hens may not have much of a claim on human feeling. But the odd thing is that as we have been learning more and more

about our animal ancestry and about our rootedness in the
world of nature, we seem to have been treating some of our
animal cousins with less and less sensitivity towards whatever
feelings they might have.

If the battery hen is a sign of our age, then it is a sign
which asks us, 'Who do we think we are?' And that too is one
of God's questions.

Sometimes, in the name of God, it has been answered
arrogantly and unfeelingly. Man is lord of creation, we are
told. Man can do what he likes with a world which has been
given him to rule. But I suspect that nowadays a humbler
note is beginning to creep in. Man is part of God's creation,
a part with special responsibilities, with unique privileges of
conscious access to God himself, but still only a part. And
therefore what we do with the rest of it is not simply ours to
decide. There has to be respect, a certain sensitivity towards
the whole fabric of life. The hopes, the legitimate hopes, of
scientists have to be set within this broader contect.

When Jesus spoke about nature, he often used it as a
parable of God's activity. Of the two parables read this morning, one was a parable of growth – the mustard seed; the
other was a parable of judgement – the harvest, the comple-
tion of God's purposes. And that is typical. God's activity
frequently has this double edge, building up and breaking
down, promise and challenge, hope and judgement. So too do
the signs of science as I read them. The promise of enormous
power, the hope for a life given new dignity and freedom, of
nature harnessed to the service of what is good and true and
wise. And then on the other hand, the judgement passed on
us by the way we use these powers; the questions asked of us,
who we are, and what we hope to be, and what our priorities
are, and how we can find our proper role in God's world, a
role constantly bungled by human failure.

But if we believe that these are God's questions, not merely
the self-doubts of anxious people, then the questions and the
judgements are themselves part of God's mercy. They are the
probing of a knife – a surgeon's knife intended to heal. God

does not bring us face to face with our sins, our failures and our limitations simply in order to cut us down to size. To see in some scientific achievements of our age the signs of God's judgement is not to be negative or fainthearted about them. It is in submitting to judgement that we are made whole. It is in acknowledging our finiteness that we can learn true wisdom. It is in humbling ourselves that we discover true power, the power of him for our sakes humbled himself to become man and gave us at Christmas time an enduring basis for hope.

11

LIVING ON TICK

When a University can boast such a galaxy of famous names it might seem unnecessary, or even impertinent, to suggest yet another. My excuse is that he is the archetype of founders and benefactors, the man who, perhaps more than any other, first laid the foundations of Judeo-Christian civilization. I refer to Moses.

The picture I ask you to have in mind is the unforgettable scene in the last chapter of Deuteronomy where this old man, who had seen so much, endured so much, and struggled so hard to weld a reluctant people into a disciplined army, stood on the top of Mount Nebo and looked at the length and breadth of the promised land. This is what the years in the wilderness had been leading to. And God said,

This is the land which I sware to Abraham, Isaac and Jacob that I would give to their descendants. I have let you see it with your own eyes, but you shall not cross over into it.

And there Moses died. And there he was buried.

The archetypal founder looked forward to his inheritance which lay in the future; an inheritance from which he was excluded by his own integrity, and by his own deep involvement in the sins of his people. There is more than a hint in the story that Moses somehow suffered vicariously. He was identified with the generation which died in the wilderness,

This chapter was originally the University Sermon in Commemoration of Benefactors preached in Great St Mary's Church, Cambridge, Nov. 1976.

not having received the promise.

But there is not only personal poignancy in the scene. There is something deeply ambiguous about the whole notion of a promised land. In the chapters in Deuteronomy leading up to the death of Moses, promises alternate with warnings. The land which flowed with milk and honey is a land full of dangers and temptations; a land of ease and apostasy. The very fact that Moses died before he reached it enabled him to keep clear of the ambiguity. He remained the archetypal leader of a people on the move.

Not so those who followed him. Their story revolves around the question – how is it possible to receive an inheritance without being corrupted by it? How is it possible to combine the advantages of a settled order, with the stimulus of being kept on the move? These are basic Old Testament themes. And they extend beyond it. It is not fanciful, I believe, to compare Moses on Mount Nebo with Jesus on the mountain of temptation. The temptation story is in any case full of echoes from Deuteronomy. Like Moses, only more so, Jesus 'saw all the kingdoms of the earth and their glory' – and turned away from them.

And the Church? The ambiguity of its inheritance runs right through history, and haunts us still. It is unfair to condemn the Church as sweepingly as Dostoevsky did, when he claimed that it had deliberately and consistently surrendered to the temptations which Jesus rejected. We have an inheritance, and nowadays it is too easy to feel guilty about having great possessions – whether in a church or in a university; too easy to pay lip-service to a great tradition and to inherited glories, as on an occasion like this, while inwardly feeling that at least some elements in them are an embarrassment and a constraint. But equally it is fatally easy merely to accept their benefits unthinkingly.

This is where the image of Moses on Mount Nebo is so potent. The promised land was no delusion. Yet it was not for Moses. I am reminded of a saying of George Macdonald: 'I do not think that the road to contentment lies in despising

what we have not got. Let us acknowledge all good and
delight that the world holds, and be content without it.'[1]
Moses did not despise the promised land. Indeed his whole
life had been directed towards it. But he was content to die
outside it.

It is this kind of acceptance, and yet holding back, this
restraint which does not despise the object of its desires, this
combination of yes and no, which lies at the heart of the
religious attitude to life.

It is not only Moses who sets his seal on it. Jesus, as we
have seen, made the same kind of renunciation. The incarnation itself presented for us a kind of divine restraint – a
scaling down to human limitations. 'Being in the form of God
. . . he humbled himself, taking the form of a servant.' In the
fulness of divine power, he stood back. Love shows itself as
much in what it does not do, as in what it does.

Religious restraint can easily be caricatured as a species of
cowardly negativity in the face of life's opportunities. Indeed,
the very title for this series of sermons, 'Living free', seems to
imply that openness and expansiveness are the main virtues
to be cultivated. My own title 'Living on tick' is meant to
indicate that those who live free often do so at somebody
else's expense. But more seriously than that, it is intended to
point to the general question with which I started: How can
we receive our inheritance without exploiting it or being corrupted by it? or more particularly: What kind of restraints
are appropriate in a society where freedom, growth, expansion, the fulfilment of human ambitions, the enlargement of
human aspiration, have become almost unchallenged norms?
I am not thinking so much of externally imposed restraints
as of inner attitudes, the assumptions of a community.

Let me illustrate in terms of one of the largest public issues
now facing us as a nation: the nuclear power programme –
whether to expand into fast breeder reactors. On one level
this is simply a technical issue demanding the most careful

1. From C. S. Lewis, *George Macdonald: An Anthology* (Bles 1963).

assessment of risks and benefits on an international scale with all who can join in at that level. But at its heart there lies a choice about the kind of future society we want. And this is a question for everybody.

If we want assured and increasing energy supplies, if we believe that our current rate of technical expansion can continue as at present on a world-wide basis without leading to exhaustion and collapse, then we have to pay the price in terms of technical and social complexity. And the character of our society will be formed by the extremely sophisticated technology needed to secure its primary resources. Energy supplies shape communities.

If we say 'No' to the next stage of nuclear expansion, then we are saying 'No' to a great many other things as well. We avoid the technological hazards, we avoid the perils of continued expansion, but we face enormous social problems: a multiplication of the kind of insecurities experienced now, the frustrated expectations of those who find prosperity receding just when it seemed to be within their grasp. We would have to settle for what is known now in the jargon as 'the sustainable society' dependent on renewable energy resources – a society which would in the long run require of its members a quite unusual degree of inner restraint.

Here, as I see it, lies the basic choice. Over-simplified, maybe; but in the end it is a choice about attitudes and assumptions. And we do not have to look far to see where our present attitudes and assumptions are leading us. I am told that there is no truth in the rumour that a Series 4 Litany will shortly be issued by Parliament with the responses: 'North Sea oil deliver us' and 'We beseech thee to lend us some more'.

But let me bring the question nearer home. What kind of inner restraints are appropriate in the life of a university? The question may have a hollow sound at a time when external restraints are beginning to bite so hard. But I ask it as a religious question, perhaps as one of the forms in which the religious question can be still heard by members of a religious institution who fight shy of Christian commitment. How do we receive our inheritance of prestige and influence and wealth and privilege, as well as our intellectual inheritance of the pursuit of any and every kind of truth, without being corrupted by them into arrogance or irresponsibility, and without losing a sense of human limitations?

I have a particular interest in questions concerning the social and ethical responsibilities of scientists and technologists. And I know the extreme reluctance among some even to face such questions as: Are there things which, though it would be technically possible to do them, nevertheless ought not to be done? Is there knowledge which it might be too damaging to human values to attempt to obtain? A week or two ago I was rung up by a Sunday newspaper and asked to comment on what the reporter described as 'the horrific proposal' to mate apes and human beings. I told him that he had answered his question himself.

I believe it is being increasingly recognized that there are limitations, there are appropriate restraints, even at the thrusting edge of scientific expansion, which need not destroy the basic motivation and method of science to explore whatever can be explored. Where there is an acknowledgement that restraint is needed, then there is some hope of making it effective. The temporary moratorium on experiments in genetic engineering is an example of corporate scientific responsibility.

Surely one of the tasks of a university is to explore these restraints and the sense of responsibility on which they depend; to explore the old frontiers of natural moral law, despite its difficulties, not just as an exercise in the Theology faculty, but as a study relevant to everybody. Surely a major task of a university is to be sensitive to whatever it is that preserves our humanness and our wholeness.

But even this is to put it too negatively. It is to concentrate on the 'no' and forget the 'yes'. It is to ignore the ambiguity; it is to assume that we first exploit our inheritance and then have to find ways of stopping ourselves from doing so.

Christian restraint, as I have tried to suggest, has deeper, more complex roots than this. It is a form of the self-limitation of love. It entails an identification with human sinfulness and fallibility. It grows out of a sense that what we inherit comes to us, not by right, but by grace. This is why it can be nourished by thankfulness, even a relatively formal act of thankfulness like the one we are now engaged in.

This is the land. We have our inheritance. And as with Moses, the deepest wisdom is to know from whom it comes, and for whose glory it is to be inhabited.

PART THREE
MEDICAL ETHICS

12
THE CHRISTIAN TRADITION IN MEDICAL ETHICS

In its origins Christianity shared with Judaism, and with most of the ancient world, a sense of the close relationship between religion and medicine. Salvation and healing, though not identical, were seen as different aspects of the same divine activity. Thus a cure for leprosy must have its ritual expression, and unforgiven sin might lie at the root of paralysis. Jesus told his followers to preach the gospel and heal the sick, and in his own ministry did both in such a way that the one illuminated and exemplified the other (e.g. Mark 2.17). Ethical problems, like whether or not it was permissible to heal on the Sabbath day (e.g. Mark 3.1–6), presupposed that healing was not an end in itself, but must be understood in the larger context of the religious meaning of life.

Though the emphasis on direct miraculous healing faded soon after the end of the New Testament period, Christianity never lost its broad concern with health. Care for the sick was institutionalized from the fourth century AD onwards in the development of Christian hospitals, almost invariably based on monastic foundations. Early scientific medicine, in the tradition of Hippocrates and Galen, was absorbed into medieval Christendom together with many other aspects of Graeco-Roman culture. But while the religious framework of life provided a support and justification for medicine, it also tended to inhibit discovery and innovation. The growth of modern medicine from the seventeenth century onwards demanded a sharp assertion of autonomy over against its former religious associations, and for a time there was widespread Christian opposition to new medical techniques.

This chapter was originally a review article in *Dictionary of Medical Ethics* (D.L.T. 1977).

Anaesthesia, narcosis in childbirth, vaccination, contraception, sterilization, and many other procedures have all been condemned by influential Christian bodies, and some still are. In more recent years, however, there has been a greater readiness for both sides to engage in rational and open discussion of the ethical implications of various kinds of scientific advance, and claims to strict autonomy, whether scientific, medical, or religious, are being modified.

The classical Christian approach to general ethical questions has been through the concept of Natural Law, which dominated medieval moral theology, and still forms the basis of Roman Catholic thinking on these matters. The concept is usually justified in Christian terms on the basis of Romans 2.14–15, though its roots lie deeper in Stoic and Aristotelian ethics than in the Bible. It is assumed to be possible, in the light of reason, to discern the laws by which human beings should live in accordance with the given facts of human nature. These laws, it is claimed, are universal and apply to all men, though in practice they may need clarification through revelation, and reinforcement by the teaching authority of the Church.

So far as medicine is concerned, any deliberate interference with normal bodily functioning is, according to this view, a violation of Natural Law, but may be justified on one of two main grounds:

(a) The principle of totality, whereby any diseased part of the body may be removed or otherwise modified if its malfunctioning constitutes a serious threat to the whole.

(b) The principle of double effect, whereby a good action is not forbidden, even if one of its unintended consequences is evil. A sterilization, for example, which would in other circumstances be condemned, might be permitted as an incidental result of the removal of ovaries for ovarian disease.

On the basis of very general principles of this kind, often applied with great refinement, the Roman Catholic Church has maintained a consistent tradition of medical ethics, particularly in areas affecting the integrity of human life and sexuality. Where possible Catholic hospitals have been established, within which the Church's distinctive ethical principles can be upheld. Directives containing precise and detailed instructions on a wide variety of medical issues have expounded the Natural Law tradition as interpreted in Papal encyclicals and other pronouncements; the most famous recent example is the encyclical *Humanae Vitae* on the subject of contraception. A few modern Roman Catholic moral theologians, notably Bernard Häring, have recorded dissatisfaction with a tradition which, in their view, relies excessively on law, and presumes to dictate the limits of medical practice from some superior vantage point outside it. They have advocated a much more open and dialectical approach to medical ethics, in which theologians and medical workers share their respective insights and problems.

Outside the Roman tradition the approach to medical ethics has been less systematic, and prior to the mid-1950s it would have been difficult to find more than scattered references to a limited range of problems. In part this reflects Protestant suspicion of the Natural Law tradition and Roman Catholic methods of casuistry (the application of laws to particular cases). In part it also derives from the tendency of Reformed theologians to begin, not with abstract principles, but with the ethical problems raised from within medicine itself. Thus growth of interest in the subject has closely followed a period of major medical advance. Furthermore, a theology which emphasizes grace, to the virtual exclusion of law, is likely to content itself with general guidelines concerning Christian attitudes, rather than detailed instructions for Christian behaviour in specialized situations. This is part of the Protestant insistence that nothing must be allowed to stand between the believer and God, not even a system of ethics.

In its positive aspects Protestant ethical thinking has tended to concentrate on general questions about the nature of man, and the quality of a truly human life as made possible in those who have responded to the grace of God. Love, freedom, and forgiveness have been favourite themes, and earlier attempts to use the Bible as a source-book of answers to contemporary problems have largely been abandoned. Many now treat the Bible as a guide to the spirit in which problems must be tackled, an authority for the values which must be preserved, and an exploration of some of the basic issues, such as the ambiguity of human createdness and creativeness, which underlie the ethics of scientific advance.

One of the first modern attempts to provide a fairly comprehensive treatment of medical ethics within this tradition was made by Joseph Fletcher, who subsequently became well known for his advocacy of so-called Situation Ethics. He described this as a person-centred rather than a principle-centred ethic, whose main thrust is to permit and encourage all that enhances personal life and freedom. In its developed form it admits of only one obligation – to love – whose implications must be worked out in an endless variety of unique situations. As a reminder that people are more important than ideas, and that circumstances alter cases, this approach has its value, but its main weakness is that it offers minimum guidance at the very times when guidance is most needed.

Unlike other Reformed Churches, Anglicanism never wholly abandoned the Catholic tradition of moral theology, but preserved a liberalized and less authoritarian version of it. This bore fruit in the field of medical ethics in the mid-twentieth century, and a report, *The Family in Contemporary Society*, prepared by a widely representative group of experts in different disciplines for the 1958 Lambeth Conference of Anglican bishops, proved to be landmark in moral thinking. It was the first report really to exploit the method of detailed empirical study, allied with interdisciplinary discussion, in such a way that theological insights were allowed to illuminate and articulate the moral claim inherent in the subject under study, without dictating prior conclusions. A notable series of similar reports, many of them on medical topics, e.g. abortion, sterilization, euthanasia, have followed the same method. It has clear affinities with the style now adopted by some modern Roman Catholic moral theologians, which was referred to earlier; but it also stands well within the Protestant tradition of biblically-inspired sensitivity and personal choice.

The use of theological insights, rather than the deduction of moral answers from unalterable moral principles, can be illustrated by some examples drawn from central Christian beliefs. Belief in creation, for instance, can act as a reminder of creatureliness, a permanent warning against the assumption of god-like powers over life and death, or against excessive interference with the actual conditions of human life as prescribed by the natural world. The doctrine has another side, though, in that it includes the notion that man himself shares in God's creative powers, and is called to act as a responsible steward towards the world of which he is a part, yet in a measure transcends. The application of such ideas to, say, the prospects of genetic engineering could be illuminating, but requires considerable subtlety in handling a delicately balanced argument.

The doctrines of the incarnation and of salvation are fundamental to Christianity and pervade most Christian thinking. One of their practical consequences is to encourage Christians to respect human potentialities even in the most unprepossessing people and the most unlikely circumstances. The belief that human nature is potentially capable of bearing the divine image has very widespread implications, which touch every aspect of the organization of social life. It might also have a quite specific and limited application, say, to questions concerning the treatment of sub-normal children.

Conversely, the doctrine of original sin, which asserts the existence of an evil bias in all human nature, acts as a corrective to naive optimism. One of its fruits may be a certain scepticism about the ability of human beings to plan successfully for their own future; there are numerous examples of its relevance to legislation in the frequency with which liberal intentions are exploited by the unscrupulous.

Attitudes towards death and suffering are of obvious concern to medical practice. The unconscious assumption that death is the worst thing that can happen, and that suffering must at all costs be avoided, seem to underlie some excesses in modern medical treatment. Christian beliefs about life after death and the redemptive power of suffering may in the past have been used to justify unreasonable opposition to life-saving techniques, but there are valid questions to be asked from the Christian standpoint about the extent to which the pendulum has now swung too far the other way.

Contemporary discussions on the nature of health, and the social dimensions of medicine, open up interesting possibilities for the recovery of something like the biblical perspective, in which health was seen as one part of a much larger quest for wholeness of personal and social life. In fact the open-ended character of the concept of health may provide one of the most fruitful new areas for mutual exploration between doctors and theologians. The very successes of medicine force it to take more seriously questions about its ultimate aims, while theologians, whose business is with ultimate questions, are being forced by conditions in the modern world to pay as much attention to physical as to spiritual realities.

These examples of the use of Christian theology imply that its characteristic contribution to the study of medical ethics is in the indicative rather than in the imperative mood. Granted a general benevolent concern for the well-being of individuals and society as a whole, different ethical choices are more likely to reflect differences of opinion, say, about the nature and destiny of man, than differences of ethical orientation. As the New Testament itself makes clear, it is easier to obtain agreement on the command to love one's neighbour than to answer the question about who precisely one's neighbour is (Luke 10.25–37). Few would disagree with the proposition that medicine is about love of one's neighbours. But what may be done to one's neighbour for his own well-being, or what constitutes well-being, or how his claims are to be set against those of his fellows, depend upon the way in which his life is understood. And that is, at least in part, a matter of belief.

The final words, though, in a Christian account of ethics must be forgiveness and grace. This is not only because any workable ethic must make provision for failure, but mainly because part of the human predicament is the fact that many decisions entail choices between evils, and even the best actions leave many claims unmet. Finite human beings have to do the best they can. To live within the context of forgiveness and grace makes it possible to accept the inevitable ambiguities of human conduct, without relapsing into complacency or cynicism, or losing hold of the vision of some greater good.

13

HEALTH EDUCATION: THE INDIVIDUAL'S PART IN THE GOOD LIFE

There is an elusiveness and ambiguity about the phrase 'the good life' which is peculiarly tantalizing for those whose job it is to plan for other people's good. Its religious overtones might suggest that theology should have something special to say about it, and no doubt this thought contributed to the invitation of a theologian to address this section of the congress. But theology has a disappointing habit of revealing that apparently simple things are not so simple after all; and 'the good life' is a case of point.

Role of Theology

Theology is concerned with our ultimate ends, with our ultimate nature as human beings, with the ultimate meaning of life in relation to God. It profoundly affects our vision of what the good life entails; but it cannot provide a blueprint of it; it cannot be allowed to short-circuit detailed discussions between experts about what policies seem on the whole to be best for the majority of people; it cannot take away from individuals the right and duty to decide what is best for themselves. This may hardly need saying in a congress with

This chapter was originally a Lecture given to the 73rd Congress of the Royal Society of Health, April 1966, and first published in the Proceedings of this Congress. Permission to reprint the Lecture has been given by the Royal Society of Health.

such a practical slant; the technical discussion of ways and means is our major concern here, and a theologian's comments on them can only be marginal. But there are times when we need to ask deeper questions about what it is all for; and this is when theology comes into its own. It carries the warning that unless experts do in fact stand back occasionally from their detailed technical considerations, they fail to see their tasks in true perspective.

There is in addition a practical reason why theology may have something to say on this particular topic. In any discussion of the relation between the individual and society, the churches have many centuries of experience, and a fine catalogue of mistakes, on which to draw.

'Health' as indefinable as 'Man'

Let us begin with some platitudes. When we speak of health education, we all have in mind a rough notion of what we mean by health; we can all point to certain obvious ills which need to be remedied; we are all aware of large areas of ignorance among the general public, the removal of which would almost certainly lead to an increase of happiness and effectiveness, and would lessen the burden on the medical profession. Platitudes of this kind need no support from religion or metaphysics. As in ethics, many of the things we do and the rules by which we live are obvious and unquestioned. It is only when we are seriously challenged, or meet a situation in which the answer is not obvious, that we are driven to ask more fundamental questions.

The definition of health, at this deeper level, is notoriously difficult. Classic definitions all made use of the notion of harmony, and these received considerable support as the nature of physiological equilibrium was gradually unfolded. But harmony and equilibrium are not by themselves sufficient. There can be normal and abnormal states of equilib-

rium. A person may reach some form of psychological equilibrium by showing physical symptoms of disease. Life itself
is an unstable process whose final end is the equilibrium of
death. Such concepts are too general and static to do justice
to the actual complexity of the relation between health and
sickness. Even words like 'normal' and 'abnormal' raise problems which cannot be solved simply by using them in a
statistical sense. Jung once wrote:

> The very notion of a normal human being, like the concept
> of adaptation, implies a restriction to the average which
> seems a desirable improvement only to the man who
> already has some difficulty in coming to terms with the
> everyday world ... there are as many people who are
> neurotic because they are merely normal as those who are
> neurotic because they cannot become normal.[1]

To try to define health in terms of mental, social and
physical well-being raises similar difficulties. Who is to decide
what constitutes a persons's well-being? If the criterion is
subjective, there are plenty of conditions in which 'feeling
fine' can be a most unreliable guide. Whereas if well-being is
treated objectively, the word tells us very little more than the
word health.

But the basic objection to all attempts to find a comprehensive formula is that they assume that we know what is
meant by man; and therefore that it is possible to specify
what is meant by healthy man. And this is precisely what
theology is concerned to deny. Man cannot be known in his
completeness, because what is most characteristic of man,
what seems to distinguish him from the rest of creation, is his
openness to a spiritual reality transcending himself. Man is
most human when he is reaching up beyond himself, when
he is creating, imagining, exercising his freedom, stretching
the bounds of normality. Martin Buber, the Jewish philos-

1. *Modern Man In Search of a Soul* (Routledge and Kegan Paul 1933).

opher, tells a story about a wise rabbi who once addressed his pupils thus: 'I wanted to write a book called Adam, which would be about the whole man. But then I decided not to write it.' In those naive-sounding words the whole story of human thought is expressed. We think we have grasped the essence of man, we think we know what is good for man; and then we discover that we have barely started to understand.

Transcending Social Normality

This is why the rebel, the non-conformist, is an essential member of society. He is the perpetual reminder that the conformities within which most people live can become a prison depriving them of the fullness of life which might be theirs. The Danish philosopher Kierkegaard was tormented all his life by the problem of how to be a Christian in Christendom; if to be a Christian is to set out on a radical adventure of faith, how can this be done in a society where everybody regards Christianity as the most normal and natural thing in the world? This is the same problem translated into religious terms.

Kierkegaard himself raises a further problem. He was one of the most profound and original of nineteenth-century thinkers, whose influence is only just beginning to be felt; yet he was a depressive. Psychologically he was a deeply disturbed and unbalanced person, whose disturbance acted as the driving force of his creative genius. There are hundreds of similar examples: Kant, Beethoven, and Blake spring at once to mind. The saints provide a peculiarly rich field for the investigation of oddities. St Francis, St Theresa, St Joan, even St Paul, might have found themselves today in a psychiatrist's consulting-room. St Catherine of Genoa suffered from acute mental and physical symptoms, probably hysterical, yet she was one of the great mystics and her life has formed the basis for one of the most comprehensive studies of mysticism. All these were people who have enriched human life, and altered the course of history, and whose abnormalities cannot be dismissed as unfortunate incidentals. By going to the very brink of human tolerance in creative achievement or mystic insight, they overstepped the bounds of what is normally called health.

These are extreme examples. But geniuses and saints are not a race apart. They reveal in an exaggerated form what is potentially true of most, perhaps all, men. And they are of particular relevance in any discussion, however mundane, of the good life.

Transcending Ethical Normality

The same point can be made in another way by considering briefly the nature of ethics. A simple-minded view of ethics considers it as a system of rules and principles which are applied to particular situations in life. Ethical theories try to reduce these rules to some comprehensive formula, some ultimate criterion like 'the greatest happiness of the greatest number', which can act as a final court of appeal when rules seem to be in conflict, or ethical judgements are challenged. The history of moral philosophy is littered with such formulae, most of them useful up to a point, all of them failing in the end to do justice to the actual complexities of human conduct. The good life cannot be defined. Ethical rules and principles are among the platitudes on which it must be based. But those who are most sensitive to the meaning of goodness are aware of obligations which no rule can specify, of possibilities which cannot be deduced from any system.

The most characteristic part of Christian ethics illustrates this. The maxims of Jesus in the Sermon on the Mount are not rules in the ordinary sense of the word. They are of very dubious application in the actual complexities of life. They consist, for the most part, of impossible demands, which have haunted the Christian conscience ever since they were uttered, and which continue to reveal new depths in the meaning of personal relations. To hear them is to be made aware of a new quality of goodness. Throughout history a few people have always tried to take them literally, and these have become symbolic figures in society, challenging the remainder not to ignore these maxims nor to assent to their impossibility too easily.

Rebellion against Healthiness

In turning from ethical to medical 'goodness' it is important to remember that the word retains its elusiveness. Our platitudes concerning health are the preliminary basis, not the content, of the healthy life. When this is forgotten, when the truth that man tries to reach beyond himself is ignored, then health can seem as boring and irrelevant as a life of mere moral conformity.

Teenage rebelliousness no doubt has many causes. Deliberate infringements of the rules of health, like taking drugs for 'kicks', or smoking too much, or failing to wash, probably take the form they do partly as a result of social accidents. But a significant feature of our age is the extent to which such rebelliousness is extolled as a virtue. Drug-taking is not universally condemned; responsible writers have defended it as a means of extending aesthetic awareness. Shaggy and seedy-looking young men become popular heroes. Smoking retains its appeal despite all the factual propaganda against it. Even a harmless word like 'clinical' has begun to acquire slight sinister undertones. It is hard to resist the conclusion that for a considerable section of the population, overmuch concern with health and hygiene has become a bore.

Rebelliousness is not confined to these matters, of course. This is a very small part of a much larger picture. Implicit in these infringements is the perfectly sound belief that health

is not an end in itself, that healthiness only has value insofar
as a person has something worth living for. And therefore the
boredom and sense of frustration which can lead to drug-
taking, or promiscuity, or many other socially undesirable
forms of behaviour, or perhaps even to that infuriating unwillingness to make use of all that the health services can offer,
have their roots deep in those ultimate questions about the
purpose of life which are the proper concern of theology.
When human life is narrow and circumscribed, when human
beings are treated as if they are all too easily understandable,
there is an inevitable reaction, either in the form of active
rebellion or passive rejection.

Health only a relative value

The practical consequences of this for those professionally
engaged in the health services are not for a theologian to
specify in any detail. The important point to remember is
that all scientific, medical and technological advances have
an ambiguous value. They can be used either for the enrich-
ment or for the impoverishment of human life. Every gain in
understanding, every plan to increase efficiency, can either
set people more free from material necessity, or make them
feel more insignificant. The only safeguard against domina-
tion by our own techniques and discoveries is to be quite
clear that they have a relative, not an absolute, value.
    The value of health is relative to the purposes which indi-
viduals have for their own lives. Health is a means to fullness
of life; but it is not an end itself; it is not even an essential
condition for a worthwhile end, as the achievements of many
sick people demonstrate. To stress this may seem like a return
to the realm of platitude, which we considered at the start.
Nevertheless platitudes of this kind are worth repeating
because every human institution has a tendency to think of
itself as being of absolute value; and this is especially true of

institutions whose aim is to promote human welfare. Purity of intention is no guarantee against the danger of empire building, as the churches have ample reason to know.

There is in fact an inherent element of frustration and disappointment in trying to plan for other people's good. The more comprehensive the plan, the greater are the chances of reaction against it in the name of what may appear to be irrational individuality. The most recent and obvious example of this is, of course, the plan for the fluoridation of water supplies. To recognize the inevitablity of frustration is not the same as accepting it meekly; but it can serve to restrain those who might be tempted to elevate a technique of relative value into an absolute necessity out of sheer annoyance.

Parallels with the experience of the churches

Theological reflection about the nature of man can help to set these frustrations in a wider context, and make them more bearable. In fact theology can help even further. One of the striking features of our modern society is the way in which the health and welfare services have taken over many of the functions formerly exercised by the churches; also, though this is not so commonly recognized, they have inherited some of the churches' problems. The sub-title of this symposium, 'Them and Me', points straight to one of the perennial themes of Christian ethics, summed up in the question: How is it possible to serve people without patronizing them or making them dependent? Perhaps the characteristic Christian answer to this may be of some use, even though there is little sign yet that the question is being seriously asked outside its Christian context. The Christian answer is in two parts; first it points to the way in which Christ served humanity by becoming a man among men; secondly it states that service can only avoid being patronizing insofar as it is rooted in worship. Neither of these insights can be applied directly to the health services, though they might apply to individuals within them. But it might well be that these insights have secular equivalents. If the secular equivalent of worship is respect, then Christian experience might remind us that those who seek to serve the public should first of all respect them.

Christ's service of humanity may seem a little less directly relevant. But nowadays one of the ways this insight is finding practical expression within the churches is in the breakdown of the barrier between clergy and laity. It is not unreasonable to suggest that one of the secular equivalents to this could be the breakdown of the barrier between doctors and patients, or between government servants and their clients. Some doctors and civil servants seem to cultivate an almost papal aura of eminence and remoteness, and are inclined to make pronouncements, like preachers from their pulpits, from six feet above contradiction. They follow the example of the medieval clergy in refusing to discuss technical matters with the laity for fear of disturbing their simple faith. So long as this attitude persists, and there are signs that it is already on the wane, the opposition between Them and Me must remain irreconcilable.

The service of humanity requires that we should stand among humanity, and address our fellow men, not as Them nor as You, but as We.

14
SOCIAL ATTITUDES TOWARDS THE SEXUALLY-
TRANSMITTED DISEASES

Historically there seem to have been three main social attitudes towards the classic venereal diseases, attitudes which reflect in part the state of medical knowledge about them, and in part general assumptions about sexual behaviour. These have in turn influenced the preferred medical approach. I shall call these approaches –
1. Legal compulsion
2. Moral persuasion
3. Moral indifference.

Legal compulsion

1. Legal compulsion goes back a long way. It is possible that an Act of 1161 forbidding brothel-keepers to keep women suffering 'the perilous infirmity of burning', may be the earliest attempt to legislate on the subject in this country. The most famous, or infamous, piece of legislation was the Contagious Diseases Act of 1866, which provided for the compulsory examination and treatment of prostitutes in certain ports and garrison towns. The opposition to this Act, which was eventually repealed in 1886, did much to focus attention

This chapter has been reprinted from *Crucible* Oct. 1975, and based on a paper originally read to a Royal Society of Medicine Conference on Sexually Transmitted Diseases and published in their Proceedings.

on the wider social problems of prostitution, and on the rights of women.

The assumption behind this legislation was that the root cause of the spread of the venereal diseases was prostitution, and that preventive measures should be concentrated on those most at risk, i.e. the armed forces. Similar assumptions seem to have underlain Defence Regulation 33B, which was introduced in 1942 and lapsed in 1947, and has been described as a 'panic wartime measure', designed to protect servicemen. This was again vigorously resisted on the grounds that it seemed to condone prostitution while taking away some of the prostitutes' rights.

The last attempt to introduce legislation in Britian was in 1968, when a Private Member's Bill sought to revive the wartime powers of compulsory contact-tracing. By this time the climate was entirely different. Prostitution was scarcely mentioned in the debate. As a subsequent *Times* leader put it, the diseases were now more likely to be 'caught from acquaintances rather than prostitutes'. The Bill was withdrawn after the Government spokesman had argued that compulsion would be ineffective anyway, and would merely make contact-tracing more difficult.

The lessons to be drawn from this part of the story seem to be that compulsion is unlikely to succeed unless there is a relatively restricted class of persons to whom it applies, and in these circumstances it raises serious questions about individual rights. However, if moral opinion were to change so radically that confidentiality was no longer an issue, the objections to compulsion would lose some of their force, and it would be possible to treat the diseases in the same way as any other notifiable condition. I shall return to this point later.

Moral persuasion

2. Moral persuasion has traditionally been the main non-

medical weapon against the diseases, but there has often been confusion between two distinct motives underlying it. There have been those for whom the moral motive has been primary, and who have regarded the prevalence of the venereal diseases as an index of the moral health of society. Eradicating them by adopting stricter standards of sexual morality has been urged on the grounds that these standards are good in themselves, and therefore ought to be upheld with medical support. Sometimes the conclusions have been drawn that it is socially dangerous to remove the deterrent effect of the diseases, but responsible moral opinion has usually managed to avoid overstressing this point. Thus as long ago as 1924 the COPEC Commission on Christian Social Morality dismissed fear as a means of countering sexual promiscuity, and wrote:

> What is needed is not a mere unwillingness to perform the act, but a moral repudiation of it. . . . To be satisfied with saying 'Avoid this, or you will suffer from it', is to stimulate ingenuity to find a means by which the consequences can be avoided and the act enjoyed. [1]

Prophetic words!

The other motive for using moral persuasion has been medical. It has been argued that the medical problem can only be solved insofar as the social, and by implication the moral, problems underlying it are tackled. There was an interesting example of this approach at a BMA Conference held in 1964 for young people. The over-whelming emphasis in a very wide-ranging discussion was on the need to change behaviour. However, the explicit reason for calling the Conference was not to discuss promiscuity as such, but to consider means of preventing the spread of the diseases.

Both motives, of course, frequently combine, especially in education work. In a paper written in 1970 on 'anti-V.D. education', Dr Dalzell-Ward made the point that 'education

1. COPEC Commission Report, vol. IV.

regarding venereal disease cannot be considered apart from education for mental health and personal relationships'. He went on to express the hope that it would be possible to 'fashion a new educational policy based on sound scientific principles, rather than upon empiricism or the mere arbitrary application of personal judgement'. [2] I find it fascinating that science, empiricism and mere arbitrary judgement should be thought of as the only alternatives. But the whole paper is interesting in that it spells out very clearly the moral dimension of the problem, and wavers between making this primary, and sticking to the safe, scientific ground of dealing with proven ills.

Awareness of the dual motivation of the moral approach may have made some doctors increasingly hesitant to use it. Among the general public there are very large numbers who still think of venereal diseases as shameful, more shameful probably than the conduct which spreads them; and there are strong lobbies which still use V.D. statistics as an index of moral corruption. On the other hand, the very strength of these feelings may be counter-productive, in that careful professional attempts at moral persuasion can seem to lend weight to moral attitudes of a much more extreme kind.

In 1971 a West Indian nurse was subjected to a routine test after returning from a holiday abroad, was accused of having contracted V.D., and was promptly dismissed by the Birmingham Regional Hospital Board. Admittedly the Board apologized when the nurse was subsequently found to be suffering from yaws. Nevertheless the whole incident seemed to symbolize a condemnatory attitude which many in the medical profession no longer wish to be associated with. And this, I suspect, is one of the reasons underlying the third approach I shall describe – moral indifference.

2. A. J. Dalzell-Ward: *Forward planning in the United Kingdom for anti-V.D. education.* Brit. J. Vener. Dis. (1970) 46: 159.

Moral indifference

3. I do not believe that the majority of people professionally concerned with medical and social problems share as a personal attitude the sort of moral indifference expressed by the teenager who said: 'I cannot feel guilty or ashamed about having gonorrhoea because I have done something completely natural like just to sleep with somebody. . . .' I want to suggest, however, that professional attitudes have changed radically in the last few years, and that professional moral indifference is a fair description of a very wide-spread approach.

The Office of Health Economics Briefing on the Venereal Diseases, issued in October 1974, expresses the change very succinctly:

> Attempts to control sexual behaviour, preventing promiscuity and so limiting the chances of infection spreading . . . are unlikely to be successful, and may today be thought absurd by those to whom they are directed. This area is so complex that would-be educators who try to change the population's sexual behaviour may even influence it in a manner which is the reverse of that which they intend.

The handout accompanying a BBC programme for teenagers on V.D., broadcast in November 1974, illustrates the same tendency. The six page pamphlet is entirely medical in content, and the only hint that there might be other aspects of this problem is contained in a single sentence at the end: 'Needless to say, the factual approach of both the programme and these notes does not assume that values held by many teachers and students concerning sex before marriage and casual relationships are to be dismissed or rejected.'

Some campaigners put it more forcefully. Thus Germaine Greer, in an article in the *Sunday Times* (February 1973) wrote: 'It's time V.D. was socially accepted', and countless teenage magazines spread the gospel of sexual liberation of which

V.D. is an inevitable, but scarcely troubling, side-effect.

Professional moral indifference has great advantages in a social climate where actual moral indifference in sexual matters is becoming more common, and where moral uncertainties are deeply felt even by those who have no liking for promiscuity. Indifference eliminates fear and guilt. In a less guilt-ridden situation the problem of confidentiality would not loom so large, contact-tracing would be easier and, as many now suggest, the venereal diseases could take their place among other genito-urinary complaints without any complicating moral overtones. 'Stop moral posturing', says the reformer, 'and treat the problem as one aspect of everyday personal hygiene. The moral emphasis may have had its value when methods of treatment were less successful, but is irrelevant now.'

I hope I have not caricatured this attitude, but it seems to me that it is not confined to the venereal diseases alone. The Family Planning Association has produced some blatant examples of moral indifference. Some of its literature seems so obsessed with the single aim of eliminating unwanted babies that virtually any sexual behaviour is condoned provided it is 'responsible' in the limited sense of not being reproductive.

Despite the attractions of this approach, moral convictions are not so easily by-passed. Neutrality or indifference are themselves moral attitudes, and what may have been adopted as a professional stance very rapidly becomes interpreted as a personal moral recommendation by those towards whom it is directed. Moral indifference conveys the message that in this sphere moral considerations are of no account.

Indifference and tolerance

Since indifference is frequently confused with tolerance, it is vital to distinguish between them. Indifference says, 'I don't care'. Whereas tolerance says 'I do care, but I recognize your right to differ.' Indifference ceases to use the language of right or wrong. Tolerance uses moral language, but uses it humbly and in a spirit of readiness to hear another point of view.

The danger I foresee in our present mood of moral indifference is that a medical profession, which for good practical reasons wants to avoid moral complications, may be unconsciously legitimizing all sorts of undesirable social practices, under the guise of being tolerant.

This process whereby one person or group legitimizes another person's behaviour is still not widely appreciated, although there are obvious and well-known examples. Crowd behaviour is a case in point. The crowd in some way gives permission or sanction for acts which in other contexts would clearly be recognized as wrong. An American study called *Sanctions for Evil* analysed the sort of permissions given by society which led, in full flower, to the atrocities of Vietnam.[3] Moral indifference about V.D. may seem insignificant by comparison. But my point is that its effects are not neutral; they may be much greater than we think.

A concern for whole persons

Another facet of the same problem is the curious irony whereby, just at the moment when so much of the emphasis in modern medicine is on the treatment, not of diseases, but of whole persons in their social context, the moral dimension is in danger of dropping out. Not from medicine as a whole, of course. There has surely never been a time when medical ethics has flourished so profusely, or the medical profession been burdened with so many difficult ethical choices. However, the focus of attention has been on the ethical problems which are, as it were, internal to medicine, rather than on the personal moral standards of patients, and the social forces which mould them. I wonder, though, whether a profession

3. N. Sanford and C. Comstock, *Sanctions for Evil* (Jossey Bass Inc. 1971).

which takes seriously its concern for health in the broadest sense of the word, can afford to remain neutral in matters which deeply affect growth in personal maturity, and which influence prevailing social assumptions about something as central to life as sexual behaviour.

The alternative to moral indifference need not be censoriousness, nor the attempt to apply moral persuasion of a kind whose motives, as I suggested earlier, can be questioned. Personal conviction allied with tolerance is a healthier mixture than either of these; and I therefore very much hope that members of the medical profession will not come to believe that in a puzzled and morally divided society, the right thing to do is to keep quiet.

Convictions expressed with tolerance and understanding create a climate in which there can be honest and open debate, but where nobody doubts the seriousness of what is being discussed. In such an atmosphere, those who look for moral guidance may find it; whereas those who reject it, need not be shamed into neglecting the medical help they need.

It would be going too far beyond my brief to try to spell out what kind of convictions might be held, and how in practice they might be expressed. May I suggest as a starting point, however, the phrase used a moment ago – 'whole persons in their social context'. Morality, as well as medicine, is about wholeness. Moral insight begins as we consider individual actions in relation to a whole life and in the broadest possible context. Religious morality widens and changes the context by the perception of a spiritual dimension. But any morality worth the name must point the individual beyond his immediate concerns and gratifications and limited horizons, and help him to see the kind of life he is making for himself and for others.

To open up such questions, even in a medical setting, is the first step towards showing that convictions matter. Nor can it be claimed that to do so is an alien moral intrusion. If my argument in this paper is sound, such questions also have an essential place in good medicine.

15

CONTRACEPTIVES FOR CHILDREN

Any Church leader finds himself bombarded from time to time with literature about the moral health of the nation. If he has doubts about its accuracy, fairness, or wisdom, and makes no response, he will be accused by some of cowardly silence and failure to give a moral lead. If, on the other hand, he accepts it at its face value and makes the right denunciatory noises, he will reinforce the suspicion that Church leaders are too readily tempted to jump onto bandwagons, and are swift to condemn from some vantage point well above the level of established facts.

It was in response to this familiar dilemma that a group of Church leaders in the North East encouraged the formation of a small working party to look into a specific moral and social problem on which they had been asked to comment – namely the supply of contraceptives to adolescents below the age of 16.

The working party contained two medical officers, a senior nursing officer, a family welfare worker and a member of the Family Planning Association, all with considerable experience in the family planning field. In addition, there was a circuit judge, three teachers, a probation officer, a pharmacist and three clergy. All had responsibilities within a single urban area, and though the group was convened under Christian auspices, its membership was not confined to practising

This chapter was originally published in *Crucible*, Jan. 1977, and is a personal summary of the discussions in a working party convened by the Social Responsibility officer for Cleveland.

Christians. The notes of its discussions were privately circu-
lated among interested parties, and what follows is a personal
interpretation which does not have the authority of the working party as a whole, though it reflects the spirit and content
of its findings.

The overwhelming impression was that hard facts about
teenage sexual behaviour are not easy to obtain. The statistics
of abortions among under-16-year-olds in England and Wales
show a steady increase from 552 in 1968 to 3,243 in 1974, and
there is a corresponding but slower increase in maternities
which, by 1970, represented almost exactly half the pregnancies. In the urban area under consideration, which has a
population of just under half a million, 10 per cent of all
births were outside marriage in 1971, and a more recent
survey showed that in the under-20 age group the proportion
of conceptions outside marriage was 70 per cent. In 1974, 69
girls under 16 were known to be pregnant; 22 were reinstated
in school after birth or termination, and about 50 were attend-
ing clinics during the period January to October. The medical
officers estimated that there must be about 100 girls under 16
in the area who were sexually active, but the subjective
impression of the teachers was that the problem is much
larger than these figures indicate.

Some members of the working party believed that the sexual proclivities of teenagers had not changed greatly with the
passage of time, and that the figures could be explained in
terms of the lower age of puberty; the fact that sex is now
more openly discussed has meant that sexual adventures are
better publicized and may be taken further than in previous
generations. These members were sceptical of alarmist claims
about wide-spread moral decline, and were inclined to look
sympathetically at teenage moral insights in terms of which
sexual intercourse was regarded merely as 'a nice thing to
do'. The moral and emotional dividing line was seen as running between responsible and irresponsible pregnancy, and
even more clearly between responsible and irresponsible
parenthood.

Other members doubted whether the level of sexual interest and activity remained unaffected by social influences, and tended to interpret the statistics as evidence of a higher degree of sexual arousal. Sex was described as a fertile ground for self-deception, and adolescents were seen as especially vulnerable to peer-group and commercial pressures and the sexual expectations of contemporary society. On the whole, these members regretted the sexual inducements and opportunities now offered to teenagers, and the Christian teachers in particular commented on the personal tragedies they had witnessed, and the lack of support they had experienced from many of their colleagues.

It was noticeable that whatever meagre evidence was available was likely to be interpreted by members of the working party in the light of their own moral convictions. However, all agreed that there were problems, and all found it helpful to examine their stereotypes of each other's attitudes. Those in the Family Planning service were sensitive to the criticism that they might be creating a problem rather than meeting a need. They felt under attack by those who saw them as part of the 'permissive society', whereas their intention was simply to do a useful job among those who would be unlikely to go for help to anyone suspected of being censorious. Clergy, on the other hand, wanted to live down their reputation of having all the answers and being swift to condemn, but found it difficult to convey the idea that having convictions about right and wrong was compatible with a receptive and caring attitude towards those in trouble. Teachers and parents confessed to feelings of helplessness in the face of moral confusion and social pressures which were hard to resist, and even some of those who knew what moral stance they wished to adopt found it difficult to defend their position.

The fact that the working party met at all was felt to be of benefit, and its main conclusion was that those who are professionally concerned with these problems need to relate to one another and share their perplexities.

With the provision of free family planning advice and con-

traceptives through the National Health Service, a major part
of the work of the Family Planning Association has been
taken over by the State. Many former members now continue
their work through the Health Service, while the Association
itself has shifted its emphasis towards sex education, and in
particular publicity concerning the availability and use of
contraceptives. 'Grapevine', an offshoot of the Association,
recruits young people to make contact with members of their
own age group in schools, sixth form colleges, clubs and pubs.

We found it difficult to obtain reliable information about
Grapevine, and were warned by a former member to interpret
their statistics with care. In principle, the idea seems a good
one. There is a clear need for reliable information about
sexual matters, and the young might seem better placed to
provide this for their contemporaries than those who are
regarded as authority figures. Nor is Grapevine confined to
sex alone. It is claimed that 50 per cent of the calls received
through its telephone service relate to problems of loneliness.
However, there is a disturbingly high rate of turn-over among
its recruits, and one who spoke to us described her frustrations
in trying to establish anything but the most superficial contact
with those to be helped. The counselling job she was trained
to perform was, in her experience, impossible in the casual
setting in which she was expected to work. She saw this as an
organizational difficulty, but some of the working party interpreted it as an inherent deficiency in the concept of the organization itself. Sex education through casual encounters not
only isolates it as a problem area, but also runs the risk of
creating needs and anxieties in the minds of those who have
been buttonholed. On the other hand if, as is claimed, Grapevine has identified and is trying to meet a genuine need, there
is a clear obligation on those who disapprove of its methods
to provide some alternative. The scope and style of what is
already done through schools, youth services, churches, etc.,
needs further scrutiny.

The fact that contraceptives are now so easily available to
young people through slot machines or over the chemist's

counter means that any prohibition on their use under the age of 16 would be ineffective, even if it were thought to be desirable. The main area of discretion left to medical advisers, apart from general sexual counselling and educational activities, is whether or not to prescribe the pill. We therefore looked at some of the legal, practical, and moral implications of doing so.

Legally the situation is somewhat obscure. The law does not directly forbid the supply of contraceptives, or giving advice about their use, to persons under 16. But in theory a doctor who prescribed the pill for a girl knowing her to be under that age, might be charged as an accessory to the offence of unlawful sexual intercourse committed by her boy friend. It is very unlikely, though, that such a charge would succeed; indeed one judge has already expressed in public his, admittedly somewhat idiosyncratic, mind on the subject, in following the principle that the interpretation of the law must take account of changing moral values.

It is possible that a doctor who carried out a physical examination on a girl under 16 without parental consent might be charged with indecent assault under section 14 of the Sexual Offences Act 1956, but there are inherent improbabilities against any parents seeking this kind of publicity for their daughter.

On the whole, therefore, it seems that legal sanctions against the medical profession can be discounted, though the matter has not yet been tested in the courts.

Individual doctors working in the Family Planning service obviously differ in their approach to under-age clients. One, who was a member of our working party and has children of her own, described how she made fairly searching enquiries into the family background, relationships and aims, ambitions and future plans of girls who came to the clinic without parental knowledge. She also pointed out to clients the social dangers of oral contraceptives, in changing the expectations of boy friends. It was her opinion that some of the girls who came to her and who had not yet had intercourse but felt that

they might soon be in a position of risk, were behaving respon-
sibly, and had weighed up carefully the pros and cons of
continuing a relationship with a boy who was increasing his
demands. Some attempt might be made to put another point
of view, but in the end the girls would not be sent home at
risk of returning six weeks later for abortion referral. This
doctor felt that by the time patients came to clinics they were
almost always committed to sexual activity, and that she
could therefore only deal with the symptoms, not with the
underlying social causes.

A memorandum from the Department of Health and Social
Security, dated May 1974, advises members of the Family
Planning service mainly on the legal implications of accepting
under-age clients, and only has a brief mention of counselling
'as an adjunct of contraceptive services'. This reinforced our
impression that the doctor whose work was described in the
previous paragraph went further than most in trying to help
young people face the implications of their behaviour, but
even she felt severely limited in what she could do.

The dilemma was put to us – how can those who work in
this field be effective helpers, and yet remain faithful to the
standards which they accept in their personal lives? All social
workers have to cope with role conflicts, but this particular
one is heightened by the fear that the non-judgemental attitude of those who give advice on sexual problems may itself
be one of the social causes of the problems. There is also the
element of challenge to established values in the sexual mores
of many young people, there are claims that we now live in
a morally pluralist society, at least so far as sex is concerned,
and there are insistent voices declaring that 'the contraceptive
revolution' has not yet been taken seriously by the traditional
guardians of morality. All of which puts considerable pressure
on those whose professional stance would in any case encourage them not to interfere in what are said to be purely personal decisions.

Or are they? Perhaps the heart of the dilemma lies here, in
the degree to which sexual behaviour, suitably safeguarded

against pregnancy, can be regarded as 'purely personal' by society at large, even in the case of adolescents in whom society still has an educucational interest. In our present state of uncertainty about the long-term consequences of different patterns of sexual behaviour, it would seem foolish to accept the 'purely personal' argument at its face value, quite apart from more specifically Christian considerations about the nature of sexuality.

The working party was unable to agree on the extent to which the moral convictions of helpers ought to be allowed to impinge on their clients. It saw that at times too sharp a distinction could be drawn between professional non-judgemental attitudes and the stereotypes of moral censoriousness. A counsellor with positive ideals may be in a better position to care and respond creatively to another's confusion, than one who is as confused as the person they are trying to help. Furthermore, though professional social workers rightly regard non-judgemental acceptance as an essential preliminary to any worthwhile relationship with a client, the fact is that people are not scientific objects who remain what they are, independent of the relationships in which they stand. A relationship with a counsellor, be it never so accepting, is always to some extent changing the person who is accepted, even if only by seeming to legitimize their present behaviour.

It may be useful to distinguish between the acceptance of another person and the affirmation of what they are. To affirm another person without question may simply tie them even more securely into the whole set of social circumstances and confusions which have led to their trouble in the first place. On the other hand the selective affirmation of those aspects of a person's character or way of life, which represent what they have it in them to become, may provide a constructive way of dealing with their problems. This does not entail imposing ideals on them in a judgemental way, but drawing out from them what the counsellor's own moral vision reveals of their potentialities.

The alternative is to allow the whole question of moral

values to go by default, in the name of liberalism and professional integrity and objectivity. But it would be ironic if, just when in many other professional fields there is a growing awareness of social responsibilities, those who deal with very human and intimate problems should feel bound to ignore moral considerations.

Perhaps the time has come when those who have moral convictions should be less afraid of making them known. We are repeatedly warned that young people, trying to find their way sexually, are put off by heavy-handed moralism, and this is why some well-intentioned propaganda may fail so disastrously. The alternative, a kind of tolerant caring, a continuing attempt to deepen moral insight, is much more demanding on those who practice it. And this is one reason for recommending that those who have to deal with these problems should be offered the support of multi-disciplinary groups.

16

EUTHANASIA

Attitudes towards euthanasia reflect and are influenced by attitudes towards death. For Christians, faith in the resurrection is central. It not only expresses what they believe about the ultimate fate of those who die, but it symbolizes and gives a basis for the style in which they believe they ought to live. 'Whoever loses his life will find it.' This is a paradoxical summary of a way of life which finds its fulfilment and vindication in the death and resurrection of Christ.

In Christian thought, therefore, death is not the worst thing which can happen to a person. It is an experience through which people pass, and is potentially of extreme importance in crowning a lifetime of surrender into the hands of God. The ideal kind of death, according to this point of view, is one in which a conscious surrender can be made in faith. 'Father, into thy hands I commend my spirit.' The words of Jesus on the cross echo an ancient Jewish bedtime prayer; they represent a way of dying which is given added significance by the belief in what followed. But though consciousness, dignity, and ultimate willingness are important factors in such a death it remains essentially a surrender, something experienced rather than something done, something accepted rather than something chosen. Thus while Christians have glorified martyrs, and have seen the martyr's death as in some sense the apogee of faith, they have persistently abhorred suicide as the supreme instance of faithlessness.

Permission to publish this chapter has been given by The Royal Society of Health. It was originally a paper, entitled 'Euthanasia: a Christian view,' presented at a conference of The Royal Society of Health, Dec. 1973, and originally published in the RSH journal, Vol. 94, no. 3, June 1974.

The right to die

Such a bald and dogmatic statement cannot begin to do justice to the range and subtlety of Christian thinking about death. It may at least serve, however, to pinpoint a distinction which is fundamental in any discussion of euthanasia. The belief that death is not be feared but is at times to be welcomed as a friend, underlay the 1965 Report *Decisions about Life and Death* produced by the Church of England Board for Social Responsibility. Its authors argued persuasively for the view that patients who might otherwise be subjected to a battery of sophisticated medical techniques designed to preserve a bare minimum of life, ought to be allowed the right to die. It was recognized that particular decisions might be extremely difficult, but the general principle was clearly stated, namely 'that in a given case, medical treatment should extend so far and no further'. A variety of arguments, some religious and some not, can be used to point to the same conclusion, but the fundamental Christian ground was the one already stated; death is not the final disaster, and therefore it is better both for the patient himself and for the medical staff concerned to accept it with good grace.

Suicide

In sharp contrast to this readiness to let hopeless cases die, is the widespread Christian belief that to take positive steps to help them to die is both socially dangerous and morally wrong. This belief rests in the last resort on the other element in the Christian attitude towards death, namely that it is God's business not ours, and that to take the power of life into our own hands is to deny our status as creatures. Such thoughts have not prevented Christians from taking such powers in judicial and military contexts, but it could be argued that there is a difference between making public decisions of this kind as a matter of social necessity, and an individual making a personal decision about the limits of his own life. Be that as it may, the fundamental basis of Christian opposition to suicide has always been that it implies a denial of the love of God who can redeem and so make bearable even the most hopeless situation, and a denial of his rights as the ultimate Author of man's life. Euthanasia, as an instance of suicide by proxy, falls under the same condemnation.

In an earlier Board for Social Responsibility Report, *Ought Suicide to be a Crime?* (1959), it was argued that although there were strong religious reasons for wishing to discourage suicide, there were not sufficient social grounds for continuing to think of it as a criminal act. There may be rare instances in which a person plans his own suicide with the deliberate intention of benefiting others, but more commonly it is not a premeditated act at all. Indeed, the overwhelming trend of recent medical and social studies has been to demonstrate the irrelevance of criminal law in this context. The fact that the law was changed in the Suicide Act 1961 owed not a little to Christian initiatives.

Such liberalization of the law concerning suicide, however, has not entailed a corresponding change of attitude towards euthanasia. Voluntary euthanasia, by which is meant the conscious deliberate decision to end one's life in certain medical circumstances, falls within that small category of suicides which the law was intended to forbid before the large psychopathological element in normal suicide was fully recognized. It is not illogical, therefore, to support a change in the law concerning suicide while rejecting legislation which would permit euthanasia.

Passive termination and euthanasia

So far I have been concerned to show that the two contrasting attitudes I have described, a readiness to let die and a refusal actually to take life, both have their roots in the Christian theology of death. For convenience, I refer to passive termination and euthanasia. I recognize, of course, that there are other arguments besides Christian ones, which can be deployed for and against both of them, but my aim in this paper is to explore whether there is anything distinctively Christian to be said about these matters, hence my assumption throughout that the Christian categories I am using have a proper validity.

If, then, such a contrast can be entertained at least in theory, we need to ask whether it can be applied in practice. Arguments in favour of euthanasia frequently blur the distinction, and it is not uncommon to find pleas for the merciful release of those who are artificially maintained in a so-called vegetable state, being used to support legislation which would permit a doctor positively to kill a patient. In terms of what is actually done or not done at the bedside, it may be that there is a very fine dividing line between passive termination and euthanasia. There is, as someone has said in this context, a difference between 'doing something' and 'doing nothing', and perhaps this is a sufficient guide in practice; however, where the question at issue is whether or not a resuscitation device should be switched off, it is hard to be precise even about this.

Further complications

Furthermore, the situation is complicated by additional uncertainties.
1. When forms of treatment are used which may have the effect of shortening a patient's life, the procedure is often justified morally on the grounds that the primary intention of the treatment may have been to relieve pain or distress, and that death has been a secondary consequence. To some this

seems like hypocrisy. Others argue that there is an important practical difference between adminstering a treatment, however potentially lethal, and administering a drug which has no beneficial effects apart from killing a patient. Admittedly we are once again in the realm of fine distinctions, but the fact that there may be borderline cases does not invalidate the broad contrast between euthanasia and alleviating treatment.

2. In such discussions it is often assumed that we know clearly what is meant by death. This is, however, yet another dividing line which has been blurred by medical advance. When a person has been resuscitated and perhaps may have suffered irreversible brain damage, or when a person, say, has been in a deep coma for a long time and shows no signs of recovery, in what sense is it still proper to go on treating them as if they were still living persons with all the rights of persons? And what is the transition point beyond which we only show them the residual respect due to corpses? Traditional definitions of death, and hence of euthanasia, have become increasingly irrelevant in such circumstances. It would be possible in theory to abandon the standard physical indications of death, and to search for some which related more closely to the cessation of personal life. Complete absence of communication might be one such sign.[1] Yet who really knows what kind of personal life is still present in those for whom communication has become impossible? Is a doctor who administers a lethal drug to such a patient killing him, or merely taking appropriate action to stop the functioning of lower parts of the central nervous system in somebody who is already dead? Whatever the answers to these questions, and so far there seem to be none, it is clear that there is a limit to the precision with which normal terms can be used.

3. Euthanasia of the kind recommended by its main proponents, is assumed to be voluntary. Passive termination may

1. Since this paper was written, a definition of 'brain death' has become widely accepted.

well be allowed in cases where a patient's previous wishes are
not known, although presumably every effort is made to discover from relatives what these might have been. But an
essential part of any legislation designed to permit euthanasia
would be an elaborate procedure for discovering and record-
ing a potential patient's wishes before he was overtaken by
the state in which euthanasia might be thought to be desirable. On the face of it this seems clear and reasonable, provided we assume that people's wishes remain constant whatever state they are in. Can we be certain of this? Some old
people who at an earlier stage may have expressed an abhorr-
ence of old age show an extraordinary tenacity in clinging on
to life when they are reaching the state of senile dementia
themselves. It may be that those who voluntarily opted for
euthanasia in their moments of strength would turn out to be
the sort of powerful characters who would be consistent to
the end. But most human beings claim the privilege of being
able to change their minds, and may well do so even if they
have no means of expressing that a change has taken place.
In short, the word 'voluntary' may turn out to be as ambiguous as the word 'death'.

Clear guidelines

In a situation bedevilled by so many practical and theoretical
uncertainties, doctors have to rely on their personal judgement when confronted with particular cases. The broad distinctions mentioned at the beginning of this paper may provide general guidelines, with or without their Christian
backing. The validity of the general principles is not under-
mined by the fact that they may be difficult to apply with
precision. Nor does the fact that they can be expressed, as
here, in explicitly Christian terms mean that they rest on no
other foundation. Where, for instance, I have referred to
respect for the limits which God has set, it might be equally

possible to refer to respect for life or for human personality. and come to much the same conclusions. It must be admitted, though, that for some of those who advocate euthanasia the desire to respect human personality is given as one of the main reasons for allowing people to die while their person-alities are still intact. Some Christians, in fact, have taken up this part of the argument and have claimed that a conscious and active putting of oneself into the hands of God is pref-erable to a prolonged and degrading surrender accompanied by progressive disintegration of the personality. This is to give an unusual twist to the word 'surrender', however, and on the whole the traditional arguments against suicide have proved stronger. Respect for life, personality, and the claims of God have been interpreted in their straightforward sense as ruling out euthanasia.

R. M. Hare has some perceptive comments on the value of generally accepted broad principles of this kind in a situation where the exercise of personal judgement is highly complex:

> Doctors would do well, having adopted some fairly simple set of principles which copes adequately with the cases they are likely to meet, to dismiss from their minds (at least when they are doctoring) the possibility of there being further exceptions to their principles. For doctors, like all of us, are human, and if once they start thinking, when engaged on a case, that this case might be one of a limitless and indeterminate set of exceptions to their principles, they will find such exceptions everywhere. There may be – in fact there certainly are – cases in which soldiers ought to run away in battle. But if soldiers were all the time asking themselves whether the particular battle in which they were fighting might be such a case, they would all run away every time. The temptation to special pleading is too great. A doctor once said to me in connection with the proposal to allow euthanasia: 'We shall start by putting patients away because they are in intolerable pain and haven't long to live anyway; and we shall end up by putting

them away because it's Friday night and we want to get away for the weekend.'[2]

Legislation

Legislation to permit euthanasia would in the long run bring about profound changes in social attitudes towards death, illness, old age, and the role of the medical profession. The Abortion Act has shown what happens. Whatever the rights and wrongs concerning the present practice of abortion, there is no doubt about two consequences of the 1967 Act:

1. The safeguards and assurances given when the Bill was passed to have a considerable extent been ignored.

2. Abortion has now become a live option for *anybody* who is pregnant. This does not imply that everyone who is facing an unwanted pregnancy automatically attempts to procure an abortion. But because abortion is now on the agenda, the climate of opinion in which such a pregnancy must be faced has radically altered.

One could expect similarly far-reaching and potentially more dangerous consequences from legalized euthanasia. It would entail a conscious public abolition of the, admittedly blurred, dividing line between active killing and passive letting die. At present, those who cross that line, or who operate in its vicinity, can do so in full awareness that there are general principles about not taking to ourselves the powers of life and death, which remain valid even when their precise application is vague. The effect on long term public opinion of any serious breach of these principles, particularly as applied to fully developed human personalities, would be incalculable.

On the analogy of the Abortion Act we might expect a gradual softening of the stringency with which the regulations

2. *Personality and Science*, ed. I. T. Ramsey (Ciba Foundation), p. 92.

were applied. But far more serious would be the fact that for the old and the ill euthanasia, whether they wanted it or not, would now be an option. Unrealistic feelings of uselessness, the desire not to be a nuisance, unwillingness to face the problems of old age, would all combine to put pressure on those who were reaching a stage in life when they were easily influenced to prefer a quick way out.

Some might welcome this picture. But for a Christian who sees death as God's final action in a human life, it is worth the effort of trying to maintain fine distinctions within our present practice, in order to prevent ourselves from creating such a society.

17

EXPERIMENTATION ON HUMAN BEINGS

In 1851 a certain Doctor Waller published the results of some 'epoch-making' experiments on syphilis in the course of which he had inoculated otherwise healthy patients with the disease, at times allowing it to develop to an acute stage in order to demonstrate the symptoms better.

It is a far cry from this sort of irresponsibility, which was not all that uncommon even up till the early years of this century, to our present sensitivity on the subject of experimentation, now being extended to include a new look at animal experiments after a hundred years' experience of the Cruelty to Animals Act. So far has the pendulum swung the other way that some researchers are seriously worried that important research projects may be hampered. And they wonder at the lack of proportion between extreme concern for individual patients' rights, and the tolerance of gross inefficiencies in medical practice and the far greater, and less justifiable, risks run by patients who enter hospitals for normal treatment. I have heard an enthusiastic Professor of Medicine claim that most discussion of medical ethics is trivial, that it is individualistic at a time when our major problems are social, and that in any case those who benefit from modern medicine have a positive duty to allow themselves to be used as research subjects as a way of repaying their debt to previous generations.

Be that as it may, modern research practices are so hedged around with safeguards, from the prior approval of Ethical Committees, to the stigma involved in publishing work later

This chapter was originally published in *The Franciscan*, Jan. 1977.

thought to be unethical, that there is a case for saying that the whole matter is now under control, and there is no need for non-specialist authors or journals to interfere! But the old platitude about the price of liberty being eternal vigilance remains true, and it is therefore important to keep the issue on the agenda, if only to preserve the present balance. There is a constant pressure in any kind of research to do the slightly more daring investigation, to explore the limits of what is permissible, and to rest in general comforting beliefs about the good sense and high social responsibility of the medical profession. Fine – provided that there are others, not so involved, who are sensitive to the issues and can flash a few warning lights.

The essence of the ethical problem under consideration is how to find the right balance between the possible harm a patient might suffer through being an experimental subject, and the possible benefits which might accrue from a particular piece of research. This is a difficult equation, because both sides contain a large element of guesswork, and the most creative research usually arises out of vague hunches which are hard to evaluate in terms of a balance sheet. As in any scientific study, there is a great deal of routine work whose benefits are fairly minimal and which only impose trivial discomforts or inconveniences on the patients who are the subjects of it. It poses no particular problems to Ethical Committees which realize that without it researchers could not be trained, and the big advances might never take place.

There are other types of research, though, where the harm is not negligible and some, for example experiments involving psychological strain, where it may not even be recognized. Biopsies, which are a common means of obtaining parts of various organs for testing, can be painful, and one wonders how much additional pain of this kind it is right to inflict on patients who may already be in considerable discomfort. A request to perform biopsies on patients known to be dying of cancer was recently turned down by an Ethical Committee for this very reason. Some research may entail a substantial risk, as in a recent project testing the effects of heroin; the choice facing an Ethical Committee in such circumstances is highly complex, and is likely to include personal estimates of the degree of competence and responsibility of the researcher and the general value of his work. This is one reason why it may not be very helpful to try to lay down general rules about where to draw the line.

There is, however, a widespread recognition that the more a patient is likely to benefit, now or at some later date, from the results of research done on him, the greater the liberties which can be taken. At one extreme, research and treatment may be indistinguishable. Indeed, it would help towards a more realistic relationship between doctors and the public if all treatment was seen as, to some extent, experimental.

At the other extreme, there are experiments done on patients, which bear little or no relationship to the reasons why they are in medical care, and from which the only personal benefit will be a sense of satisfaction at having done something useful. Christians, in particular, will not wish to under-rate this motive. In fact there are shining examples of those who have been able to come to terms with illnesses or disabilities by volunteering as experimental subjects.

In a field where risks and benefits are so uncertain, a good general principle is that nobody should be asked to expose themselves to unnecessary harm unless they have freely consented to do so. The vital importance of free and informed consent is emphasized in all ethical discussion about human experimentation, and in all official memoranda on the subject. It provides an obvious and essential basis for most of the things which human beings do to one another, all the more necessary in the medical context because patients go to doctors trusting that their own interests will be the doctors' main priority. A suspicion that this was not so, and that other interests were being served behind patients' backs, would do much to undermine public confidence in the profession.

In practice, though, 'free and informed consent' is not nearly such a straightforward concept as might appear. In a situation where 'doctor knows best', and where the technical issues may be quite complex, it is doubtful whether many patients know or care about what they are consenting to. There is evidence that even experimental subjects who work in para-medical disciplines find it hard to appreciate the risks to which they are being asked to expose themselves. There is also the long tradition of medical mystique which has made open and honest communication between doctors and patients the exception rather than the rule. The cards are heavily stacked, therefore, against those who might be tempted to withhold consent if they fully understood what was involved.

Nevertheless the need for informed consent acts as a certain safeguard, which might be considerably strengthened if nurses as well as doctors were involved in the process of obtaining it. Patients tend to talk to nurses much more freely about their worries than to doctors, and nurses have much more opportunity to assess what they are really feeling, or the discomfort they may be experiencing. Chaplains, too, may be useful mediators, provided they are trusted by researchers to appreciate the complexities and the importance of research. A Chaplain who could make himself sufficiently knowledgeable to serve on an Ethical Committee might occupy a very strategic role.

The regulations about consent have a major deterrent effect against experiments on children and others whose consent cannot be readily obtained. This is undoubtedly a wise precaution, though awkward for paediatricians. It illustrates the way in which a general principle, though unsatisfactory and ambiguous in practice, can nevertheless have firm applications.

This brief paper only skims the surface of a vast subject, on which the literature is steadily growing. The most magisterial work is a thousand-page volume[1] by Jay Katz, an American lawyer, who was set on his course by a study of the

1. *Experimentation with Human Beings*, Russell Sage Foundation, N.Y., 1972.

Nuremberg proceedings against the Nazi doctors. The comparative recentness of that example, and sinister revelations in our own day about medical compliance in torture techniques, may serve as a reminder that beneath the surface of the apparently marginal problems to which moralists give their attention, larger issues may be lurking. Come to think of it – my Professor of Medicine might be persuaded to see that what he dismisses as trivial could be acting as a kind of ethical prophylactic.

18
THE ETHICS OF CLONING

A squat grey building of only thirty-four storeys. Over the main entrance, Central London Hatchery and Conditioning Centre, and, in a shield, the World State's motto, Community, Identity, Stability. . . .

It is interesting that the opening words of *Brave New World* should be on the subject of reproduction control. For those who have nightmares about a science-dominated future, nowhere is there a more sensitive area than in the things which affect the inner constitution of human beings.

Aldous Huxley went on to describe 'Bokanovsky's Process', a technique for budding fertilized cells, up to a maximum of 96, and applied only to those destined to become lower grade humans, the gammas, deltas, and epsilons. Cloning, as now understood, is not budding in quite the sense in which Huxley imagined it. But the effects are much the same, the production of more or less identical copies from a single original organism without the combination of male and female genetic material. Gardeners do it all the time. Huxley simply extended the idea to people.

A student in the class being shown around the Central London Hatchery was bold or stupid enough to ask where the advantage of the technique lay. The reply went straight to the heart of the book. 'Bokanovsky's Process is one of the major instruments of social stability.' In the world state of

This chapter was originally a Lecture delivered to the London Medical Group at Charing Cross Hospital, Jan. 1979.

the future identical people would work identical machines, united in a world brotherhood of slavery.

I quote *Brave New World*, if only to demonstrate that the idea of cloning is not new. The possibility of actually doing it to animals, however, did not begin to hit the headlines until the 1960s, and the technique of transplanting nuclei into unfertilized eggs, which is the present basis for cloning, is even more recent than that. J. B. S. Haldane, in an essay written in 1963 and entitled 'Biological Possibilities for the Human Species in the next Ten Thousand Years' assumed that the cloning of human beings would be commonplace, and concentrated his attention on the difficult question of whom to clone. He opted for elderly geniuses, who would then devote their declining years to teaching their replicas, but made an exception in the case of dancers and athletes who, he said, should be cloned young. He added on a more humble note: 'On the general principle that men will make all possible mistakes before choosing the right path, we shall no doubt clone the wrong people.'

Haldane's speculation was typical of the period, and was taken up in Rattray Taylor's *The Biological Time Bomb* (1968), which foresaw sinister possibilities in some unscrupulous despot creating an invincible army of clones. There matters rested until in 1978 a sensational and allegedly factual account of human cloning by an eccentric millionaire brought the whole subject back into the limelight. The scientific world was horrified; the book in question is now the subject of legal action in the U.S.A., and the whole story will no doubt shortly be revealed as the science fiction which most responsible commentators have claimed it to be.

Reality is much less exciting. Frogs can already be cloned by nuclear transfer. The nucleus of a cell from the parent to be cloned is placed in an unfertilized host ovum, which then develops into an offspring identical with the single parent. Mice have been cloned by a different technique involving prolonged inter-breeding. Work is proceeding on rabbits and no doubt on other animals as well, and as the procedures become standardized and simplified there will almost certainly be commercial pressures to clone successful farm animals, and perhaps race horses, as a means of propagating proven good stock. Cloned laboratory animals are useful in providing standardized material for genetic research, and the techniques employed in cloning may well have a spin-off in cancer research. Cloned human beings are not as yet a practical possibility and, science fiction apart, it is difficult to see what the advantages would be in trying to produce them. Emotional and financial restraints are likely to operate powerfully against substituting a highly dubious and complicated method of human reproduction for one which operates to most people's satisfaction without the need for scientific conjuring tricks. The slow, and still to some extent surreptitious, acceptance of artificial insemination, in spite of the fact that it meets a distressing human need, is evidence of the general unwillingness to interfere too readily with fundamental sexual processes.

Nevertheless one can never tell what human folly will do. 'Try all things possible' is for some scientists part of their scientific creed. It is therefore worth asking what the ethical issues would be should anyone decide to do the experiment of producing a human clone.

The first reason for caution is simple ignorance of what the wider effects of human cloning might be. The greater the awareness of the extreme complexity and subtlety of the self-regulating mechanisms which keep biological systems in balance, the greater the reluctance to substitute conscious planning for natural processes. This caution is what its name implies, an invitation to pause, not a recipe for stagnation. But there have been enough disasters caused by premature scientific attempts to go against the grain of nature to make one suspicious of radical interference with something as basic to life as sexual reproduction. Nobody knows what social, psychological, and economic changes might result from the development of a simple and reliable technique for choosing the sex of children. The effects of a similar freedom to create clones would be even less predictable, and the advantages which might accrue highly dubious.

Of course, it can be argued that this general caution applies only to the massive application of cloning techniques, not to the few discreet experiments which might be enough to satisfy scientific curiosity. The unpredictability, however, applies as much to individuals as to populations. We are as ignorant of the feelings of a potential clone as we are of the effects of populations of clones on society. Here again the example of Artificial Insemination by Donor can serve as a warning. There is still no agreement about the desirability of telling children conceived by A.I.D. that this was their origin, or about the psychological consequence of doing so. The problem of identity, of knowing who one's parents were, is not to be brushed aside. So what would be the effects of knowing that one was a replica?

I have already touched on the second major ethical issue, that of identity. Fiction writers have tended to assume that clones would be identical in all respects, and would therefore be dubious about their individuality. In fact this is no more likely than in the case of identical twins. It is even possible that clones could be less like one another than identical twins, because it it not known yet whether the transplanted cell nuclei are the sole determinants of development, or whether the characteristics of the unfertilized ovum also make a difference. Cloned frogs certainly look alike, but there is no means of telling at present whether the similarities are more than skin deep.

Even granted an identical physical makeup, there still need be no problems concerning individuality. Our personal existence as individuals, though it has a physical basis, does not depend on the fact that we have a unique genetic inheritance. Individuals are unique because each has a unique history, makes unique choices and has a unique self-understanding. Personality is the product of personal relationships with other people. Ultimately, from a Christian point of view, each of us has a unique existence and a unique importance, because we stand, whether we know it or not, in a unique relationship with God.

There is therefore no sound reason to believe that cloning would threaten individuality. But it might well pose some problems about relationships between members of the same clone of a kind already experienced by some identical twins. I foresee greater problems, though, as I have already suggested, in terms of the relationship, or absence of relationship, with parents.

It would seem to me morally suspect deliberately to produce children with no hope of normal family life. Obviously there are plenty of instances now when this happens unavoidably, which is why the moral sting must be in the word 'deliberately'. There is also a large area of ambiguity covered by the word 'normal', and I am not assuming that the pattern of father, mother, and child is the only possible one for healthy development. There are plenty of contrary instances, but in all of them the fact of natural linkage seems to be important. There are subtle questions of similarity and difference, relationship and distance, which have to be worked out between parents and children, and it seems highly probable that a cloned child would have more than ordinary difficulties to surmount.

The third ethical issue, and one which always arises in questions of this kind, can be summed up in the question, 'Who decides?' Lord Rothschild asked in 1967, 'Should everyone be allowed to clone themselves if they wish?'; to which the obvious answer is, What sort of egomaniac would want to perpetuate a replica of himself if he had any insight into his own deficiencies? And if he had no insight, would he be the sort of person anyone else would be glad to welcome in a second edition?

On a more serious level, the general question of the control of untried human powers is one on which Christians at least are bound to be sceptical. Scientific utopias have a tendency to ignore sin, and ambitious programme of eugenics, of which cloning would be an extreme example, have an especially tainted history. This is not to say that all interference with human heredity is wrong. There is clearly room for remedying some obvious and distressing hereditary defects. To pass from this, though, to positive planning for the production of desirable types raises all the issues of racial superiority in a different guise.

One of the delightful features of life is its variety. This has evolutionary importance in that the generation of variety is nature's way of preparing for an unknown future. I believe it also has religious importance in that the seemingly inexhaustible range of different life forms, and the variations between individuals, reflect something of the infinite splendour of God. Identity and stability, in Aldous Huxley's World State motto, may seem desirable in the eyes of dictators. But I trust they will remain in the realm of science fiction.

19

PROLONGATION OF LIFE IN THE DEFORMED NEWBORN

Introduction

Within the past century the health indices of the population in general and particularly of children in Britain have improved dramatically. One hundred years ago one in six of all infants failed to reach its first birthday and of the remaining five one had died before the age of 15 years. The process of childbirth was hazardous. High maternal mortality was associated with a high infant mortality rate and the population was maintained only by a high rate of reproduction. Since then many of the causes of the high mortality have been eliminated. Increased affluence, improved social conditions, conventional public health measures and the development of preventive personal health services have controlled many of them, particularly those associated with infectious disease.

The reduction in deaths from pneumonia, tuberculosis, diphtheria, gastro-enteritis and measles has moved concern for infant survival from the first year to the first week of life. The perinatal rather than the infant mortality rate now acts as the prime indicator of child health. Overall reduction in childhood mortality has had a profound effect on population growth, family size, and reproductive behaviour. Age at marriage and family size both have fallen. Small families are now planned in the confident expectation of an uneventful preg-

This chapter was originally the report of a working group set up by the Northern Regional Health Authority under the author's chairmanship.

nancy, a safe delivery and a normal child.

Although small, risks to the infant do remain. The current perinatal mortality rate of over 22 per 1,000 is largely due to fetal loss from anoxia, congenital abnormality and problems related to low birth weight. In addition, these same problems result in some surviving babies being handicapped for the rest of their lives.

Although low birth weight and cerebral anoxia may be prevented in future by even more effective obstetric care the factors responsible for congenital abnormalities are less amenable to modification. The aetiology of some abnormalities is partly understood – those associated with thalidomide and rubella on the one hand, or chromosomal and biochemical abnormalities on the other. However, the most numerically important, the malformations of the central nervous system, remain largely unexplained although it seems probable that a mixture of adverse influences, some of which are intrinsic and some environmental, is involved. For example, myelo-meningocele and anencephaly are known to occur more commonly in social classes III, IV and V, to older parents, in families with an existing history of congenital abnormality, and in particular geographical locations. In these, as in many congenital abnormalities, prevention is impossible at present, and society, the professions and the parents must deal with the situation when it arises.

Until the last two decades few ethical problems existed in relation to these newborn babies. The majority of those with severe abnormalities or who had suffered damage during delivery died during the newborn period or in early childhood. Advances in medical treatment, antibiotics, and the development of anaesthetic and surgical techniques applicable to the newly born have changed this situation. Many children who would previously have died survive as a result of treatment to a life of dependence, deformity, and disability. It is for this reason that an ethical dilemma arises. Should deformed newborn babies who can never be restored to normality be actively treated, or should treatment be withheld in the knowledge that although the majority will die a few may survive with increased disability?

The general ethical problem may be broken down into several practical issues. The first is simply whether doctors have a moral obligation to give all available treatment to such babies, or whether active treatment should be reserved for selected patients? If selection is acceptable, what factors in any individual should be considered when a decision about treatment is made? Detailed medical data relating findings during the newborn period to long-term disability are now available for some conditions and these do allow rational selection on clinical grounds. But should social factors be considered as well? Increasing information is becoming available about the social and emotional impact of conditions such as spina bifida upon the child and the family. For example, physical problems associated with the day to day management of the child are often are magnified by poor housing and financial hardship; frequent hospital admissions and out-patient visits disrupt family routine and deprive other children of parental supervision; marital relationships become strained, sexual difficulties develop and parental health deteriorates.

Another major problem is that of decision-making itself. The extent to which parents should be involved in this process is difficult to define. In the few social studies of spina bifida it was found that both parents experienced a mixture of shock, grief, and confusion during the days and weeks after the child's birth. Although explanation of the abnormality and its effects had been provided immediately, few parents were able to appreciate its implications for a week or more. Apart from those who had previous experience of a similar child few played an active role in the decision about treatment. However, although the extent of the parental contribution may be limited it is vital both that it is made and that the parents' views are sought in a way that avoids placing an impossible onus upon them.

The final group of problems relate to the management of

the child for whom no active treatment is indicated. At present the detailed management of such children varies greatly. Some clinicians feel that once such a decision has been made it is better for parent, child, and hospital staff for the child's life to be terminated as soon as possible by sedation or some other means. Others feel that such active intervention or the application of dual standards of nursing care are not right and therefore simply withhold active resuscitation, surgical treatment, and antibiotics. This latter approach means that some children survive for longer than a few days and enables the mothers of some to look after them at home for a varying length of time. We have little evidence of the emotional effects of withholding treatment from a child on either the parents or the nursing staff involved, but whether the child dies in the newborn period or survives for a longer time there is good evidence that continuing support to the parents is vital.

Medical considerations

Although there is a wide spectrum of abnormalities of the central nervous system, ethical problems occur principally in babies with myelomeningocele with or without hydrocephalus, commonly called spina bifida. The disability of these babies varies from gross mental handicap with paralysis of the legs and incontinence, to only moderate muscular weakness of the legs. The information needed in order to make medical judgements about the treatment of such babies include the aims, results, and costs of active treatment on the one hand, and the effects of withholding or delaying treatment on the other.

Active Treatment
During the past decade in a number of centres, particularly Sheffield but including Newcastle upon Tyne, a policy of

almost universal early surgical treatment for the spinal lesions and the associated hydrocephalus has been followed. This has been associated with active medical support and follow up services at spina bifida clinics. The aims of this approach were to reduce mortality, prevent further damage to the spinal cord and brain, reduce the risks of infection, and make the care of the baby easier for the mother.

This policy has been pursued long enough for the results to be clear. In Sheffield, Lorber found that it was possible to divide babies with myelomeningocele into two groups on the basis of physical findings during the first day of life. The largest group were those with initial adverse criteria: severe paraplegia, gross enlargement of the head, kyphosis, associated abnormalities or major birth injuries, or a theracolumbar lesion. In spite of very active treatment involving an average of five operations and ten weeks in hospital only 40 per cent of these survived until the age of seven years, all of whom had severe physical handicaps and only 7 per cent of whom had an IQ of over 100. On the other hand 84 per cent of the babies without initial adverse criteria survived until 7 years, 20 per cent with only moderate physical handicaps, 16 per cent with an IQ of over 100, and 50 per cent with an IQ of over 80. On the basis of these results Lorber advocated that early active treatment be given to selected babies only.

As it is only 10–12 years since active treatment of myelomeningocele became possible few children have yet reached young adulthood. The evidence from those who have, however, is that the difficulties of childhood are exaggerated in adolescence. Physical handicap, relative immobility, incontinence and in many cases intellectual handicap make independent life almost impossible.

The total cost of an active approach to the treatment of babies with myelomeningocele must be assessed, though it should be measured largely in human rather than in financial terms, both of which are difficult to do. In a number of independent studies on the effects on family life there have been consistent reports of deterioration in marital relationships, increase in the tension in the family atmosphere, and behaviour problems in siblings. The annual financial cost of treating, educating, and housing all cases of myelomeningocele in England and Wales managed in the Sheffield manner has been estimated as £3¾ million and the cost of simply maintaining each survivor as £3,000 per year at 1973 prices.

Effects of withholding active treatment
When considering the possibility of selective treatment of babies with myelomeningocele it is essential to know what happens to children who have not received active treatment at birth. A number of reports have been published recently and although the details of criteria for withholding operation and care given to the babies varied in different centres, all have shown that very few of the babies treated conservatively survived for more than one year. Thus, although conservative treatment does result in problems in the care of babies during the early weeks and months, it does not result in the survival of many babies with gross handicap.

Continuing Care
Previous policies of active treatment have led to the survival of many children with severe brain damage, resulting in a combination of major intellectual and physical disability. The majority of families are unable to make the necessary physical provisions for such children, let alone the necessary emotional adjustments. Many of them, therefore, have to be cared for in hospital and special schools.

Their disabilities may include complete or partial paralysis. If this is below the waist it is often associated with complete loss of voluntary control of both bladder and bowel, together with skeletal deformity. They therefore present a major nursing problem.

There is also a small number of children quite unable to initiate useful or purposeful movements either independently or with help. Those who are the most disabled physically also have the lowest intelligence. Such a combination results in a child with no apparent understanding of or response to his surroundings, with restless unco-ordinated movements, uttering distressing meaningless cries, totally incontinent and unable to perform any useful tasks.

Nurses often show outstanding sympathy and care for such children, almost all of whom are likely to have been rejected by their parents. Emotionally unresponsive, they require not only constant observation but also protective furnishing to prevent self-injury. Despite the loyalty they are capable of evoking, it is difficult to regard the quality of life of these children as anything but unacceptable.

The Ethical Issues

Children like those described in the preceding section pose the ethical problem in its sharpest form. It is hoped that consideration of this particular problem will help to throw light on other cases where medical factors may be different but the ethical factors much the same. For the purpose of this discussion, therefore, the kind of case in mind is that of a newly born infant with spina bifida of such severity that there are strong, well-founded, doubts that the child, if it survives at all, will ever be able to enjoy an independent and worthwhile life. It will be assumed that in less severe cases it is relatively easy to give the child the benefit of the doubt, to encourage its survival and to mobilize the resources of the family and society at large to cope with the resultant problems. While it is clearly impossible to draw a sharp dividing line between these two types of case, nevertheless for the purpose of this discussion a convenient distinction is that enshrined in the phrase 'initial adverse criteria' (see page 165). In a high proportion of cases with initial adverse criteria, the matter resolves itself since the infants die within the first few weeks after birth. But there are other cases, and these constitute the nub of the problem to be considered, where a deliberate choice has to be made by some responsible person about what to do, or leave undone.

On what principles can such a choice be made?

Some doctors have no doubt that in such circumstances it is right to relieve suffering even at the cost of destroying life. The suffering in question may be that borne by the child which may have to face a long series of painful, and ultimately ineffective, operations, and which in any case can look forward to a life of severe physical and emotional deprivation. There is also the suffering of the parents to consider, though in their case the balance sheet is more difficult to draw up. The prolonged agony of caring for a child which can never hope to achieve a normal type of existence may be much harder to bear than the sudden pain of loss soon after birth. On the other hand, some find a high degree of fulfilment in giving their love to severely deformed children, and may feel guilty if they believe they have not done everything they could. Others who feel guilt at having given birth to such a child, may need the opportunity to love it in order to work through their feelings. In other cases, a child with spina bifida can have such a traumatic effect upon a home that the distress it causes others can have repercussions on itself, thereby setting up a vicious circle of suffering. Society suffers too, if only through having to bear the cost in money, resources, and dedicated lives in order to enable such children to survive and be provided for.

When the costs are reckoned up, there are those to whom the answer seems unambiguous and obvious. Eliot Slater puts the point succinctly:

The payment in suffering in (this) group is enormous. By the time the child has reached several years of age the psychological investment in his future has been large, both for the parents and for the child. At the time when the child is born, the investment of the parents is nine months of their lives, the investment of the child himself is zero. My conclusion is that we should put first things first: prevention of suffering comes before preservation of life.[1]

Others might state their conclusions less starkly, but their priorities are no less clear. Even if Slater's final sentence is softened to read: 'the prevention of heavy suffering comes before the preservation of a low quality life', the general principle is the same; of the two traditional aims of medicine, the prevention of suffering and the preservation of life, the former carries the greater weight. It is the balance of pain and happiness, in other words, the utilitarian principle, which holds sway.

The same principle is applied in those terminal conditions in which it is widely recognized that 'officiously striving' to keep a patient alive may be an abuse of medical skills. Equally, society as a whole has now accepted that the lives of the unborn may be sacrificed in some circumstances for the benefit and well-being of their prospective parents. Proposals to legislate for active voluntary euthanasia are also on the agenda, and in the eyes of many of its advocates there is no fundamental difference between letting a patient die when his case is hopeless, and helping him to die when all the parties concerned have decided that it would be advantageous to do so.

But at this point it is worth asking what might be the long term consequence of creating a medical environment in which judgements concerning pain and happiness were the sole criteria for making decisions about life and death. Are doctors willing or able to take upon themselves the onus of deciding what condition or 'quality' of life is 'acceptable' for their patients? The present balance between the aims of medicine, though it creates conflicts and may be impossible to maintain under extreme circumstances, nevertheless acts as a safeguard against the subtle acquisition of powers over life and death,

1. From a B.M.J. Symposium on Severely Malformed Children.

which hitherto the medical profession have neither wanted
nor been allowed.

Pursuing this question a little further, we can ask whether
the utilitarian principle can be taken as the sole guide in
medical ethics, or whether there is some other principle which
needs to be held in balance with it. In fact it is interesting to
reflect that behind the two traditional aims of medicine, and
as it were supporting them, lie two broad ethical theories
both of which have been found necessary in practice to com-
plement and correct each other. The theory that ethical
decision entails making an estimate of the balance of suffering
and happiness for all those concerned in a contemplated
action, is so widely accepted nowadays as to need no further
explanation or justification. It seems natural to try to draw
up a balance sheet of happiness for a family with a deformed
baby and, in the case of the baby itself, to try to make some
estimate of its potentiality for enjoying itself or finding even
some minimum of fulfilment. On a wider social scale, questions concerning the use of medical skills, the allocation of
resources, the provision of institutions and other forms of care
and support, likewise in the end involve estimates of what is
best for the happiness and well-being of society as a whole.
On the level of social legislation there seems to be no other
fair and reasonable way of making decisions.

The other approach to ethics seems at first sight to be much
narrower and more restrictive, less adaptable to the extremely
complex circumstances in which most decisions actually have
to be made. The assertion of over-riding moral principles, for
example the principle of the sanctity of human life – or, more
generally, the principle of respect for human personality –
can seem to introduce an arbitrary authoritarian note into
the discussion which should be open and uncommitted. Yet
in fact such principles simply reflect what most people believe
to be the case about human beings, namely that they *are*
valuable and therefore their lives *ought to be* respected. It is
true that behind such statements lie centuries of Christian
teaching about the nature of man. The classic expression of

the value of human personality is contained in the Christian assertion that Christ died for everybody, no matter who they are, and that therefore in the eyes of God everybody counts. Even for those who cannot assent to their religious basis, such claims have importance. Furthermore, this approach to ethics has its supreme virtue just at the point where the other approach is weakest, namely in the attitude it encourages towards minorities.

To argue solely in terms of general happiness provides no safeguard against injustice towards individuals. A newborn child with severe spina bifida has little to put in the scales of a utilitarian balance, unless the sheer fact of its humanity is respected. No doubt in many cases such respect for its life will be outweighed by the potential misery the child might suffer and cause. But unless there is seen to be a conflict of principles at stake, not just a single principle, the gradual assumption of powers over life and death could become too easy. And the converse is also true. To assert respect for human personality, and so to preserve life at any cost without considering what in general makes human beings happy may, and often has, led to unnecessary suffering for the sake of blind adherence to beliefs.

This digression on ethical theory may help to set the specific problem of spina bifida in a broader context. The dilemma in which, say, a consultant may find himself when confronted by a particular case, has roots which go deep into the very nature of ethics. His judgement on a variety of practical features of the case will, of course, influence his decision. So will his general ideas about the kind of happiness attainable in a family with a deformed child, and his views on the degree of quality of life which he is prepared to respect. But underlying his choice, whether he knows it or not, there are other more theoretical questions about his whole approach to ethical matters.

It is possible, in fact, to think of an ethical problem in terms of a series of levels.

At the deepest level there are questions about ultimate aims

and life-styles and values. In the case of medicine, some have
been codified in the traditional aims of medical practice, and
reasons have already been given to suggest that the balance
of these should not be altered. Considerations about happiness and the relief of suffering need to be supplemented by
sharp reminders that life is sacred whether we are happy or
not. But conversely, the principle of the sacredness of life is
not to be applied woodenly as if all types and qualities of
human life in all circumstances ought unthinkingly to be
preserved.

At the intermediate level the implications of these decisions
about values have to be spelt out in general terms. What, for
instance, is this 'life' which is to be so highly respected? Are
there degrees and qualities of life so that it is possible to
specify a minimum below which efforts ought not to be made
to preserve it? The phrase 'acceptable life' recurred frequently
in our discussions, but itself raises formidable problems.
Acceptable to whom? And who has the right to decide
whether or not another person's life is acceptable? And even
if the right were conceded, in what terms could a minimum
degree of acceptability be defined?

Very severe malformation of the brain might be used as a
possible criterion on the grounds that in such cases there
could be no development of personal relationships, and hence
no apparent personal life. Except in the most extreme
instances, though, the diagnosis of such severe malformation
shortly after birth would be a hazardous business.

Other sorts of criteria, such as the likelihood of a severely
deformed child being able to live a relatively independent and
satisfying life, present even greater hazards. There is a surprising ability of seemingly hopeless cases to achieve a kind
of happiness.

There is the further point that those who seek to judge
happiness, judge it according to their own standards, usually
on the basis of half a lifetime of physical and mental normality. 'What you have never had you don't miss.' Congenitally
blind children, for example, adjust to their blindness in school

much quicker than those who have known sight and become blind.

It would appear, then, that any attempted definition of 'acceptable life' must include a very low minimum specification if it is to avoid the danger of penalizing those whose capacity for fulfilment may be small but ought not to be dismissed as negligible. It is likely also that from time to time the specification would have to be changed in the light of medical advance. Even if the cut-off point were defined as that below which no development of personal life was possible, it could not be assumed that there will always be fixed indications of when this is so.

Another way of approaching the problem at this intermediate level is through the concept of 'ordinary/extraordinary means' as used in Roman Catholic moral theology. This concept is based on the principle that although man does not possess the power of absolute ownership over life he does have the powers of stewardship. He is expected and obliged to exercise reasonable stewardship over life and bodily health. This reasonable stewardship requires him to use what are, all things considered, ordinary means of safeguarding life and health; he may take, but is not obliged to take what are, all things considered, extraordinary means.

In most instances what is an ordinary procedure from the medical point of view will coincide with what is an ordinary and therefore obligatory procedure from the moral point of view – e.g. such developed techniques as intravenous feeding, blood transfusions, use of oxygen, surgery, etc. But there may be exceptions because, in assessing the ethical issues, the concept of ordinary/extraordinary means allows elements other than the strictly medical to be taken into account. In the case of the handicapped newly-born the circumstances which can call for closest consideration are:

the qualitative element: what level of living will medical intervention offer to a child?

the hardship element: what burdens will be placed on parents by the permanent care of a severely handicapped child?

the social element: how strained are medical resources by the following of a non-selective policy?

These elements, taken either individually or collectively, can effect the distinction between ordinary and extraordinary means and, as a consequence, leave room for a policy of selection in the treatment of the handicapped newly-born. In particular, according to this concept:

given a clear issue in which death is certain and anything that can be done will achieve survival for no more than a short period (i.e. a few weeks or, at the most, months), it is relatively easy to judge that extensive efforts need not be employed to accomplish this. It would suffice to offer the basic ordinary means of food and good nursing; if the case is one in which the use of modern techniques will provide survival for the child but will only offer a future that is going to be substantially painful and/or unhappy, one can say that the techniques are extraordinary means. The parents may request them, assuming that the social element is not an over-riding consideration, but they are not obliged to make the request; when modern techniques – including repeated surgery – whilst leaving the child severely handicapped can give hope of a level of existence that will be substantially happy *for him*, they would not be extraordinary measures. He may not be able to contribute anything to society from a utilitarian point of view, but society can contribute something notable to him. It may be that if parents are left with the burden of caring for such a child, the stress will be too heavy for them to bear without the serious risk of notable disabling effects. However, one would hope that this hardship element would not be a decisive factor but that other agencies would be able to come to the assistance of the parents.

At its third, and most practical, level ethical discussion must be concerned with technical considerations of the kind which have already been making their presence felt at other levels. The definition and recognition of 'initial adverse criteria' involves the use of medical rather than ethical skills. The social implications of medical policies which might increase or decrease the number of deformed children needing institutional care need to be spelt out in financial terms. There are exceedingly difficult questions about the proper distribution of limited resources. And there are even more difficult ones, closely related to religious values, about what a society gains or loses in the long run through the amount of care it devotes to its less fortunate members.

The main purpose of this paper, however, has been to illustrate the ethical complexity of decisions which some doctors are having to make. Awareness of the complexity, the conflicts of principles, and the different levels at which choices are made, may encourage those who have to face these issues to regard any present policies as temporary unavoidable compromises, rather than as final solutions.

Summary and Conclusions

Untidy problems do not have tidy solutions. There is no simple ethical formula which can be applied unambiguously to a large class of problems. In situations where there is a conflict of principles those responsible for making decisions need to be kept aware of the conflict as a stimulus to self-criticism.

It is not incumbent upon the medical profession to treat cases in which the likely benefits of such treatment are very dubious. Thus in the present state of medical knowledge the policy of selection for the treatment of spina bifida is in our opinion justified. We believe that the list of initial adverse criteria on page 165 gives a sufficient basis for such selection, but we recognize that these criteria change and should be subject to constant scrutiny in the light of medical advance and the ethical conflict referred to above.

However, no general statements of this kind can override the responsibility of the doctors concerned to make particular decisions in individual cases.

One way of ensuring that decisions do not go by default or become a matter of routine is to devise proper consultative procedures, both among the medical staff and with parents. An advantage of such consultation is that it also provides a means of support for those involved in the decision-making and the subsequent emotional adjustments.

Infants not selected for treatment are likely to have a very short life span. We believe that there is no case for shortening it still further by any form of euthanasia.

The long term aims of medical research in this field must be to recognize the causes of these abnormalities and to remove them.

20

ETHICAL PROBLEMS OF SCREENING FOR NEURAL TUBE DEFECTS

Introduction

The era of early surgical treatment for virtually all babies with severe spina bifida has passed; most surgeons and paediatricians now agree that such intervention in the newborn period is appropriate only for a minority of carefully selected patients. However, problems remain, as some babies with severe disease survive for several months or longer. These children suffer from prolonged disabilities, repeated illnesses and operations, and their familes experience many stresses. In spite of a number of epidemiological clues, the cause of neural tube defects remains unknown, and efforts have therefore been directed towards the recognition of abnormal foetuses in early pregnancy with abortion as the remedy.

The ability to recognize severe spina bifida by examination of the alpha-feto protein in the liquor amnii has been a real benefit to mothers known to have an increased risk of bearing such a child. Many have been able to face another pregnancy with confidence, relying on amniocentesis to give early warning of a recurrence. The discovery that a raised level of alpha-feto protein in maternal blood in early pregnancy enables a further high-risk group of mothers to be identified, before the

This chapter was originally a Report by the Working Group in Current Medical/Ethical Problems Northern Regional Health Authority. Printed with the permission of *Spina Bifida* Theory (an international journal), copyright by Eterna Press, P.O. Box 1344, Oak Brook, Ill. 60521, U.S.A. (1978).

birth of an affected child, creates an exciting prospect of extending these benefits. It seems likely that if all pregnant women were to undergo a simple routine blood test, the majority of severe neural tube defects might be eliminated, with considerable savings both in terms of human suffering and in financial terms.

Screening on such a massive scale, however, would raise a number of problems, practical and ethical, some of which are discussed in this paper. In order to see them in context, the implications of a screening programme in the Northern Region are outlined.

The test involves a blood sample at 16 weeks gestation and, as the timing of this is critical, most mothers would need to make a special visit to the ante-natal clinic for it. Although a neural tube defect is likely to occur in only 3 out of every 1,000 pregnancies, an abnormal blood alpha-feto protein is probable in nearly ten times this number, i.e. in about 1,200 pregnancies each year in the Northern Region, in which there are about 40,000 births annually. These 1,200 women would need ultra-sound examination to confirm the length of gestation and to exclude twins (the commonest cause of raised alpha-feto protein); about 700 of them would then need counselling and diagnostic amniocentesis. In about 120 each year the liquor alpha-feto protein would also be raised, and these mothers would require further counselling and, if they wished, an abortion at about 18 weeks gestation.

Ethical Problems

1. Allocation of Resources
Resources available for the Health Service are finite, and so decisions about their use entail an assessment of priorities which has ethical overtones. It has been argued that the cost of introducing a screening programme is likely to be regained within three years, by saving from the medical, educational,

and institutional care at present needed for children with spina bifida, but this assertion is almost certainly too simple. Screening, even if widely used and effectively carried out, could not reduce for several years the services needed for handicapped children already born; and if it were not widely accepted, the financial benefits of the scheme would be greatly reduced.

Furthermore, a screening programme would contain many hidden costs, in addition to the obvious increases in ante-natal clinic, scanning and laboratory facilities, as well as hospital beds and staff for amniocentesis and abortion. Especially during the early years of the service, much time would be needed for counselling patients before the initial screening test, and at every stage thereafter. Effective communication between consultants, family doctors, and patients would be important and would add to secretarial costs. Details would depend upon the local organization of the service, but it is our estimate that three major centres for ultra-sound examination and amniocentesis would be needed in the Northern Region. These would have to be in close contact with local ante-natal clinics, and preferably also with general practitioners who would often be the best people to undertake the initial explanatory work about the implications of the test. All this would cost money.

However, money is not the only consideration. Whether, as has been claimed, the service were to become self-financing or whether, as its critics claim, it would be an additional burden on the Health Service, the cost in human suffering which it might relieve could be great. But so are some of the possible risks and disadvantages, and it is on the balance of these, rather than on finance, that the discussion ought to hinge.

2. Risks of the Procedure

The major risks in the proposed screening programme are easy to define, but less easy to quantify. Amniocentesis may damage the foetus or induce an unintended abortion, especially if it is carried out in units with little experience. The tests carried out on the liquor amnii are not completely reliable, and a false positive test could lead to the abortion of a normal foetus. The liquor alpha-feto protein is raised in the presence of foetuses with other, and potentially treatable, abnormalities, and until these can be distinguished from foetuses with spina bifida they also are likely to be aborted. As a result of these possible errors, a pessimistic estimate is that one potentially normal foetus may be lost for every affected foetus aborted.

On the other hand, false negative tests would lead to false reassurance, and there is the added risk that patients would interpret a negative result as meaning that no other abnormality was present. While this risk would be reduced slightly by other tests on the liquor specimens, e.g. chromosome studies, these would greatly increase the cost of the service, and introduce a further period of uncertainty for the patient concerned. Chromosome studies, performed without further reference to the patient, e.g. into Down's syndrome, might sharpen the ethical dilemma if the results became known, and it is doubtful whether such information should be made available without specific consent given beforehand.

Should all the technical problems of amniocentesis and liquor analysis be overcome, there remain the problems, both medical and psychological, associated with relatively late abortions. Patients require admission to hospital for periods of one to four days, and there are significant risks, for example cervical trauma, infection and haemorrhage, although these may be regarded as no greater than the risks of carrying an abnormal foetus to term. There are also the largely unexplored problems of guilt following an abortion undertaken on medical advice.

It is clear that the risks of this screening procedure are substantial, though not such as to make it inadmissible, provided that the highest quality of service is assured, knowledge of the magnitude of the various risks made widely available, and the effects and complications monitored carefully.

3. Personal Attitudes

Personal ethical problems associated with routine pre-natal screening centre on the fact that the only 'treatment' offered, in the event of a positive result, is abortion. For those who believe that abortion is in almost any and every circumstance wrong, the main issue is already foreclosed. For those who find no difficulty in contemplating abortion at 18–20 weeks or even later, the personal implications of screening are relatively minor. For others, who accept abortion as a regrettable necessity only when there seem to be strong reasons for it, the problems are harder.

Put at its crudest, there is the paradox of an advance in diagnosis, which enables a decision to be made whether or not to kill the patient. Of course, it can be objected that the patient is not the foetus but the mother. This would be easier to maintain if there was in fact a clear dividing line between the premature infant, on whom all the techniques of modern care are lavished, and the mid-trimester foetus which is intentionally aborted. The former is treated as if it had the full rights of a person, whereas the rights of the latter are subordinated to the interests of its mother, its family, and society at large. Abortion and infanticide may in theory be quite different, but in practice, at a late stage in pregnancy, they form two ends of a continuous spectrum. The way the actual distinction is made seems to depend less on age than on a fallible judgement about the quality of the foetus. A foetus believed to be normal has a greater chance of being treated as a potentially valuable person than one believed to be defective. Such judgements of quality may be inevitable, but it is worth stressing the fact that they are being made, and could well become more difficult as the precision and scope of pre-diagnostic tests improve.

The point is made starkly as a reminder that normal criteria about the value of advances in diagnosis cannot be applied in this instance without remainder. They lead into an area of ethical ambiguity. The advantages of tests which would undoubtedly serve to reduce anxiety, suffering, and the personal and social burden of caring for those who are seriously defective, have to be set against the fact that any abortion, and especially a late one, entails a hard moral decision. Even though tests may be routine and there may be a strong assumption that termination is permissible, in each case there is a life at stake, and it is this which distinguishes these tests from any others. In an earlier study on the ethics of selective treatment of spina bifida the point was made that the policy of selective treatment is acceptable in the absence of anything better. The same might be said of a policy which entails routine abortion. It could be acceptable as a temporary expedient while research directed towards prevention continues. Fresh medical advances constantly alter the balance between reasonable expectations of survival and unreasonable interference in the conditions and quality of the life that is lived. Policies which may be acceptable, therefore, at one stage of advance need constant scrutiny, particularly in view of the likely increase in the number of tests of which abortion will be the outcome.

For those who acknowledge that this is an area of ethical ambiguity, routine testing would give rise to a number of secondary problems. The most serious of these would be the unnecessary anxiety and distress caused to expectant mothers to whom abortion, for whatever reason, was unacceptable, and who discovered that they were among the 3 per cent recommended for further investigation after the initial blood test. This group would have their normal maternal fears of deformity greatly heightened, without having any corresponding relief in knowing that 'treatment' was available. On the other hand, 97 per cent of those routinely tested would gain some relief from anxiety, though not without risk of disappointment.

Related to these hopes and fears are questions concerning a pregnant woman's growing relationship with her child, and the possible damage to this relationship if false hopes have been aroused, or unnecessary guilt or fear engendered. Furthermore, there is the possibility that in a society where defect was being systematically eliminated by abortion, those who had slipped through the net might find themselves burdened by a sense that they were unwanted and ought not to have been born.

None of these problems may seem of much significance in comparison with the difficulties of coping emotionally with and caring for the seriously deformed. Cumulatively, however, they articulate the hesitations of those who see the long term dangers in moves towards a society in which the elimination of a widening variety of those with genetic defects has grown to seem as normal and inevitable as abortion seems today. Some degree of encroachment on the rights of every individual to be born and to receive maximum care, would seem to be justified in view of the already very large medical encroachment on the natural processes of selection and mortality. The question is, how much? And what safeguards is it possible to build into the procedures so that individual wishes are respected, and the drift towards centralized decision-making about acceptable types of human being is not allowed to develop too far?

The most obvious safeguard would be to ensure that each step in the process of testing, and not least the first step, was voluntary, and that its implications were fully explained to parents. A system of contracting-in would ensure this, but would have the disadvantage that the social classes most at risk (i.e. IV and V) are those least likely to enter a voluntary scheme, and with the greatest tendency to book late. A system of contracting-out would ensure that a much higher proportion of the population was screened, thus making the total programme more cost effective; but it could put undesirable pressure on individuals to conform, unless adequate opportunities were provided for explanation and expert counselling.

Pilot schemes under the two systems could help to determine the take-up rate in each case, and could also give experience of the problems to be met in counselling, and the resources which would have to be devoted to it. Without such experience it would be irresponsible to launch a full-scale national scheme.

Conclusions

1. Routine pre-natal screening for neural tube defects has great potential benefits, but should not be instituted on a national basis until further pilot studies have been performed.

2. A national screening programme may not save money, but should not be discouraged for that reason.

3. The high standard of skill required for ultra-sound diagnosis and amniocentesis could best be maintained by concentrating resources in a relatively small number of centres in each region.

4. Each stage of the screening process should be clearly understood as voluntary, and should be accompanied by appropriate personal explanations and counselling. The initial explanations and informed advice on the significance of the blood test should be given as early as possible, preferably before the referral to hospital.

A PERSONAL POSTSCRIPT

Those who try to think and write on the frontiers between
theology and other disciplines are in constant danger of min-
imizing the theological dimension of their thought. The effort
to say things in language which will not raise unnecessary
barriers, and which will be comprehensible to those who do
not share Christian assumptions, can easily create the appear-
ance of a sell-out to secularism.

Preaching is a different matter. If it is to be worth anything
at all, it has to be about God. The fascination of preaching
lies in the attempt to speak convincingly of God in a specific
context whose mood, atmosphere, and unspoken questions
have been sufficiently assimilated by the preacher to put him
en rapport with his congregation. This dependence on context
means that on the whole sermons do not transfer well to the
printed page; only four of them appear in this book.

As an expression of 'a working faith', therefore, the book
is unbalanced, and contains much less direct theological
assertion than I am normally accustomed to make. This personal postscript is intended to help redress the balance. I
have tried to write honestly about the internal structure of
my Christian faith.

The account is inevitably partial and hopelessly inadequate
for all sorts of reasons. Not the least of them is that often we
do not know ourselves what we believe until other people or
changing circumstances drag it out of us. But the fundamental
reason is that religion is about the unsayable – and the recognition that there *is* the unsayable is often the first and most
important element in faith.

I am a Christian because Christian language, symbolism and practice help me to express this sense of mystery, this awareness of extra dimensions of reality, in a way that gives content to it without seeming to falsify it. This is a large claim. It rests on the assumption that human beings are in some primary sense aware of the transcendent. If we are not, I fail to see what argument or secondary experience would ever be sufficient to make us aware. This is not to say that argument and philosophical exploration are useless. I am far too attracted by them to dismiss them so cavalierly. My point is simply that they help us to recognize something which is already inwardly and deeply known, rather than to construct some new vision of reality de novo.

To put it another way, God must reveal himself to us as God if we are to know him at all. There must always be some direct element in our experience of him, something analogous to our direct experience of persons, for which no amount of argument or mental construction can ever be a substitute.

The fact that some people seem at first sight to have no such awareness clearly needs explaining. It may be that, because our interpretation of this awareness is culturally conditioned, there are times when the culture of the day no longer provides easily accessible forms in which to express it. It may be that the awareness is in some ways fragile, so that sensitivity to it can be blunted by misuse or neglect. But I believe that human beings cannot for long cease to care about the transcendent, or to search for the kind of reality which constantly eludes us, without losing something distinctively human. The root of my religious awareness is thus summed up for me in words like 'aspiration', 'hope', 'longing', 'vision'. For me the constant grappling with insoluble problems, the wrestling with words and symbols to express what has only been glimpsed in odd moments, is one of the most satisfying of creative activities. If I could write poetry or paint, no doubt these would fulfil part of the same function. Beside such wrestlings much else can seem unbearably superficial and complacent.

Edwin Muir says it far better than I can:

I who so carefully keep in such repair
The six-inch king and the toy treasury,
Prince, poet, realm shrivelled in time's black air,
I am not, although I seem, an antiquary.
For that scant-acre kingdom is not dead,
Nor save in seeming shrunk. When at its gate,
Which you pass daily, you incline your head
And enter (do not knock; it keeps no state)

You will be with space and order magistral
And that contracted world so vast will grow
That this will seem a little tangled field.
For you will be in very truth with all
In their due place and honour, row on row.
For this I read the emblem on the shield.[1]

The seemingly unreal world of images, of 'toys', as he puts it, is not small or remote or antiquated. It is by his reverent use of these that he enters the real world – the world of meaning. For a Christian the toys and images of the Christian story not only are inexhaustibly rich, but provide a safeguard against mere fantasy by their rootedness in hard historical fact.

Austin Farrer got it right, I believe, in his now somewhat neglected book *The Glass of Vision*. Biblical revelation is through 'living images', which constantly grow and attain new depths of meaning by their interplay with events, and which allow the events themselves to display their divine significance. In the end the Bible has to vindicate itself by its ability to speak on this level. It still excites me to find that it does.

One aspect of the richness of the Bible lies in the diversity of images; this has the effect of making it impossible to sit

1. Reprinted by permission of Faber and Faber Ltd from *The Collected Poems of Edwin Muir*.

down and go to sleep in some finally established theological position. Thus one of its themes is the inevitablity of constant change, and its relation to the unchanging. How can the God who seems so different on different pages of the Bible nevertheless be the same God? To understand this in terms of living images is to avoid approaching it first and foremost as a literary puzzle to be dismissed by some critical device, however illuminating the criticism itself might be. It is the symbolic presentation of a paradox whose existence in relation to God allows us to keep open the options in our own lives.

Other familiar paradoxes of the Christian faith have their roots in different biblical perceptions – grace and freedom, for instance. On one level this can seem like one of those useless intellectual games in which Christians find themselves trapped, and waste their time in defending opposite viewpoints. Who gets excited now about the Arminian controversy? Yet the word 'freedom' is probably the most explosive in the world today. To be politically aware is to hear people saying, 'I want to be myself, but how can I be myself unless somebody else affirms who I am?' To be scientifically aware is to recognize the enormous limitations set on the concept of freedom; it is to see ourselves more and more in terms of what is given in our inheritance, our circumstances, our relationships, our social environment. It would be easy for different interpretations of freedom to polarize into apparently irreconcilable opposites, as has already happened at times in Christian history, and is at least partly true of Eastern and Western understandings of freedom today.

But where there is a cultural framework which allows the co-existence of apparent opposites, where paradox is permitted without being allowed to slide into mere contradiction, the possibilities of human life are enhanced and the dangers of polarization diminished. I am not referring just to a broad tolerance which says 'It doesn't matter if you disagree, because it all comes to the same thing in the end anyway.' Disagreements do matter. What people believe about freedom is of vital importance. But to grasp that our understanding of freedom may have to be paradoxical because the only ultimate freedom is that which derives from the grace of God, allows the disagreements to be faced and worked at.

My Christian faith, therefore, allows me, indeed encourages me, to hold onto opposites; and this enlarging function is part of the meaning it has for me. The Gospel is about life being richer and more varied and more complex than most of the cultural systems we inhabit seem to make room for. Scientific man, political man, economic man, and all the other stereotypes need room to breathe in terms of some other image which includes and transcends them. Admittedly, religious man has sometimes appeared even more constricted than the rest. Where religion goes wrong, it goes devilishly wrong. The actualities of church life may seem to give the lie to what I have written about enlarged vision and breadth of insight. But because it is about the fundamentals of human existence, religion is always potentially capable of breaking out of intellectual and institutional confinement. In fact it is doing so all the time, which is why many of the practical problems of church leadership lie in precisely this area – the relationship between the old and the new.

I wrote earlier that there is a safeguard against fantasy through being rooted in hard historical fact. A personal apologia is not the place for arguing a historical case, though obviously there is much which ought to be said on this topic. The question I want to pose, rather, is what does it mean to me when I claim that the Gospel has historical foundations? How am I really affected by something which is only accessible to me in history books?

History can be used in various intellectual ways – to vindicate a set of images (the cross is a valid symbol because it happened), to explain how we got where we are (church history adds depth to our self-understanding), to underline the importance of the actual and the material (incarnational theology), and many others. But the emotional impact of historicity is something other than, and more than, this kind of underguiding of intellectual positions. There is emotional security in belonging to an historical process.

In knowing my own cultural history, I know where I belong. In believing that this cultural history has some sort of universal validity, I have a means of assessing and assimilating change without being overwhelmed by it. The more fully I am aware of the currents which have shaped the past, and in particular the more I see these as illustrating the work of God, the more ready I am to face the future in the expectation that God is to be trusted there too.

To the charge that all this might be fantasy, I would answer that there is a corrective element in history, even in the deeply-felt history of a particular tradition. In the end, the continuance of a tradition depends on its ability to match the experience of actual people. The fact that Christianity has endured so long, and in so many different settings, and in the face of such massive changes in human self-understanding, and that through all these there run identifiable and centrally important threads which unite the past with the present, is to me evidence of truth. Scientific claims to truth in the end rely on the consensus of those who have taken the trouble to master their subject matter; though I recognize that there are important distinctions to be made, it seems to me that in this respect at least religious claims to truth are somewhat similar.

The faith I try to bring to bear on the practical problems with which this book is mainly concerned, is thus constantly formed and reformed through the interaction between direct experience, traditional symbolism and historical critique. There is nothing novel in this. I suspect it is how Christians have always operated. But as I said in the introduction, I claim no more than to illustrate how one fairly conventional Christian has tried to put his faith to work.

INDEX

freedom: 15, 20, 112, 188; of publication 25

genetic engineering 43, 113
genetics 6, 28
God: awareness of 186; character of action 56; of the gaps 9 ff
Grapevine 136

Haldane, J. B. S. 156
Hare, R. M. 147
health 114, 117 ff
Hick, J. 13
history 189
humility 50
Huxley, A. 155

Incarnation 56, 74, 103, 113, 123
individuality 158

Jesus, healing ministry 109
judgement of God 99 ff
Jung, C. 118
justice 82 ff

Kant, I. 26, 42
Katz, J. 153
Kierkegaard, S. 119
knowledge, godlike 54
Knox, R. 22

leisure 95
life: quality of 172; sanctity of 170
limits to behaviour 91, 105
Lorber, J. 165

Macdonald, G. 102

man, nature of 9ff, 53, 74, 99, 113, 116, 170
meaning, limitless horizon of 27
Medawar, P. 45, 47
medical ethics, progress in xiii
Monod, J. 17
moral indifference 129, 138
Moses 101
Muir, E. 187

natural law 35 ff, 105, 110
neutron warhead 88, 91
New Scientist 43, 75
normality 118, 159
nuclear weapons 69

ordinary and extraordinary means 173
original sin 113

Pannenberg, W. 26
paradox 188
pollution 68
posterity, obligations to 80
power: of God 57; technological 51
preaching 185
promised land 102
prostitution 125 ff

Raven, C. 5, 20
rebelliousness 121
Reed, B. ix
research, medical 150 ff
restraint 74, 104
Resurrection 141
risk: analysis 81, 179; of nuclear energy 65
Rothschild, Lord 159